REBOUNDING TO BETTER HEALTH

A Practical Guide to the Ultimate Exercise

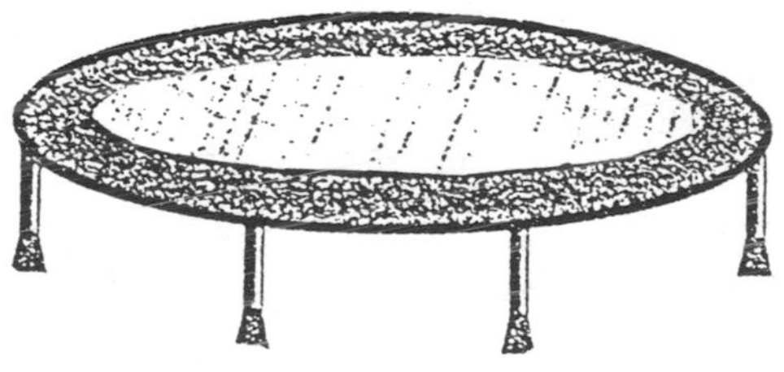

by

LINDA BROOKS
Certified Reboundologist

KE PUBLISHING

REBOUNDING TO BETTER HEALTH

A Practical Guide to the Ultimate Exercise

ISBN 0-9647265-0-5

Printed in the United States of America.

Second Printing June, 1997
Third Printing July, 1999
Fourth Printing July, 2001

Disclaimer

The information in this book is not intended to be a substitute for medical advice in any case. The author is offering information only, which is not medical advice or a remedy for any medical condition.

REBOUNDING TO BETTER HEALTH

A Practical Guide to the Ultimate Exercise

by

Linda Brooks
Certified Reboundologist

Please write to me for information on:

- Rebounders and stabilizer bars
- Personal rebound exercise programs
- Certified Reboundologist Workshops
- Seminars or speaking engagements
- Free copy of "Vital Health News" containing rebounding updates and routines, nutrition articles, and more (see subscription information on page 93.)
- Catalog of rebounding and nutritional products

Linda Brooks
The Vitally Yours Center
750 Boyce Street
Urbana, OH 43078

937-484-8206
Email: reboundvy@aol.com

Rebound exercise — effective, easy, and fun — holds a treasure of benefits for literally everyone.

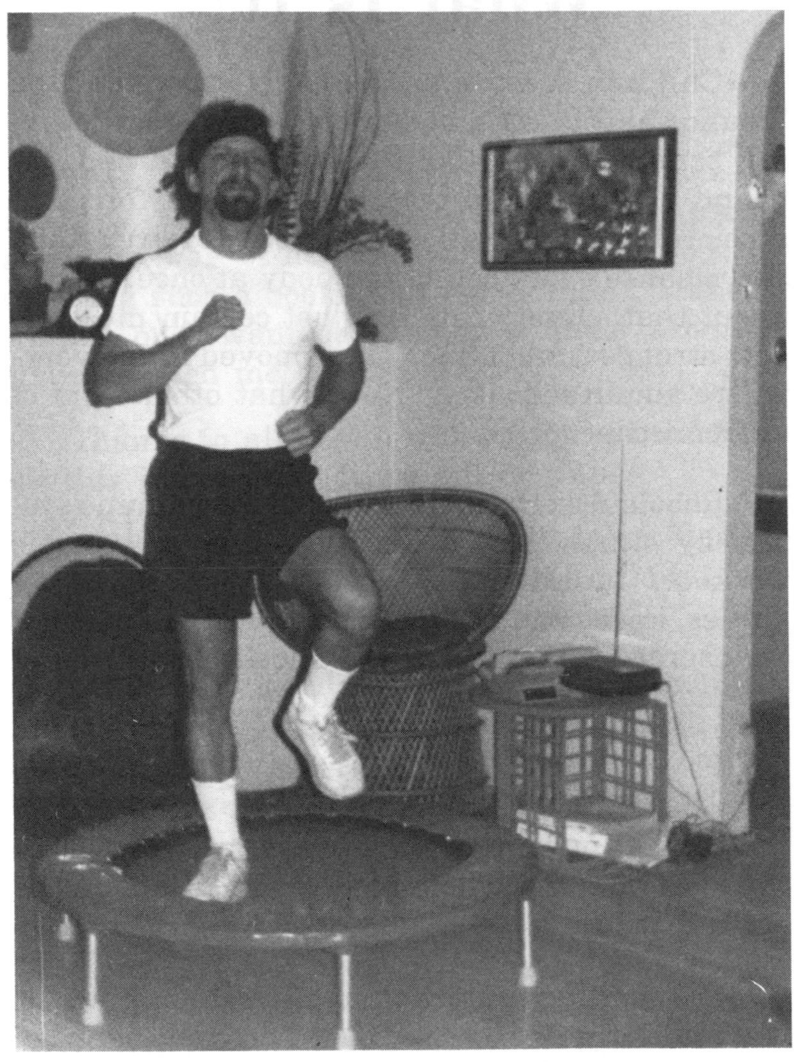

"IT IS A WONDERFUL WAY TO EXERCISE THAT IS NOT TOO STRENUOUS. IT MAKES ME FEEL VERY CENTERED AND RELAXED AFTER A WORKOUT. TIME GOES BY QUICKLY ON THE REBOUNDER."
PAUL PULASKI

CHAPTER II

How Does It Work?

Rebound exercise puts a positive stress on every cell of the body to become stronger and cleaner by the action of three natural forces on the body at once.

When you walk, run, swim or play tennis, you are constantly opposing gravity with every move. Since gravity pulls us toward the center of the earth, we can visualize gravity as a vertical force.

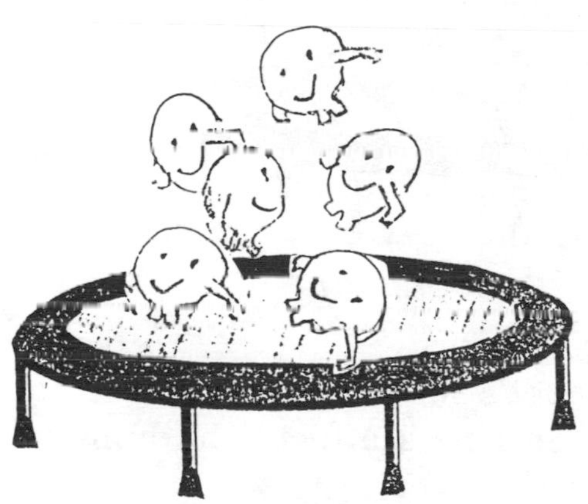

As you bounce on your rebounder, gravity is obviously pulling you down after each bounce.

Now, let's look at the other two forces involved in exercise. We start the movement with acceleration and stop with the force of deceleration. In all those exercises mentioned above, like running, the acceleration and deceleration are experienced on the horizontal plane.

Here's where the magic of rebound exercise begins. As you bounce, you are accelerating and decelerating on the same plane with gravity — vertically instead of horizontally. This is the only exercise that utilizes these three natural forces on the same plane.

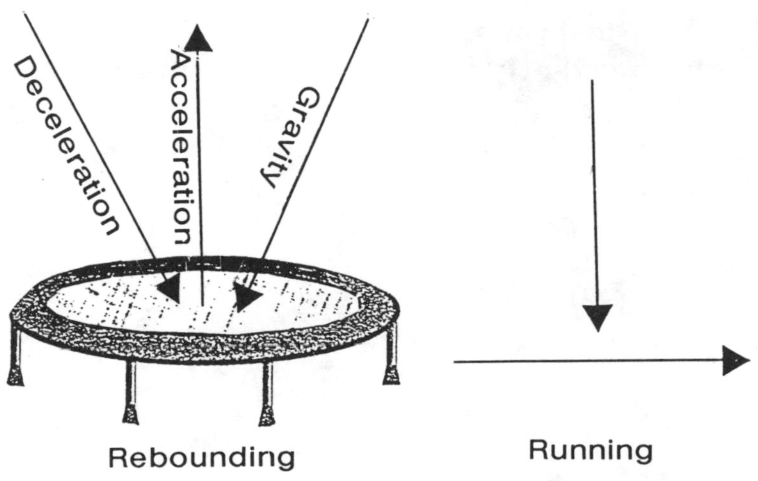

Now, let's see how the combined alignment of these three forces affects the human body.

The cells of the body know how to adjust to gravity naturally, by becoming stronger. Because of the repeated opposition of gravity, the muscles of a weight lifter get stronger because the cells of the muscle adjust to the repeated opposition to gravity.

On the rebounder, every cell of the body is being stimulated by the forces of acceleration, deceleration, and gravity. The subconscious mind doesn't know the difference between these three forces. It computes them as three gravities and reacts to this triple force by telling the cells to adjust positively.

As you bounce on your rebounder, your cells experience a gentle squeezing at the bottom of the bounce, pulling toxins from the cells, while stimulating them to become stronger.

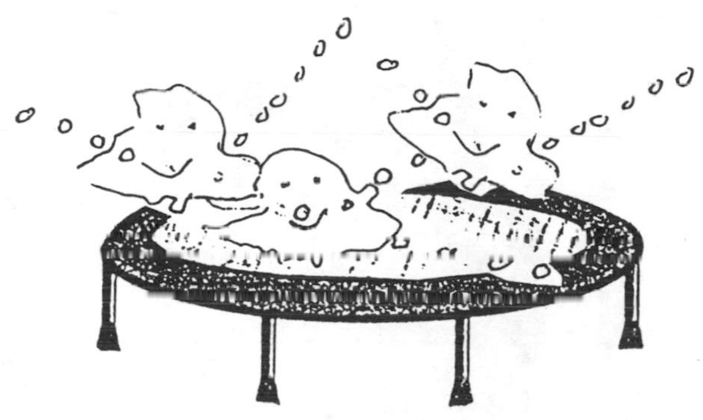

That's a simple, not-so-complicated explanation of how rebounding works. There are hundreds of other benefits. A study by the University of Oklahoma shows that because the mat of the rebounder absorbs 87% of the shock of the bounce, this exercise is safe and healing to all cells of the body.

As a matter of fact, N.A.S.A. has studied rebound exercise and declares it to be 68% more efficient than regular jogging. This is the <u>only</u> exercise that will stimulate the cells of your internal organs, veins and arteries as well as bones and muscles, while increasing circulation and flushing the lymphatics.

Have you exercised your spleen today?

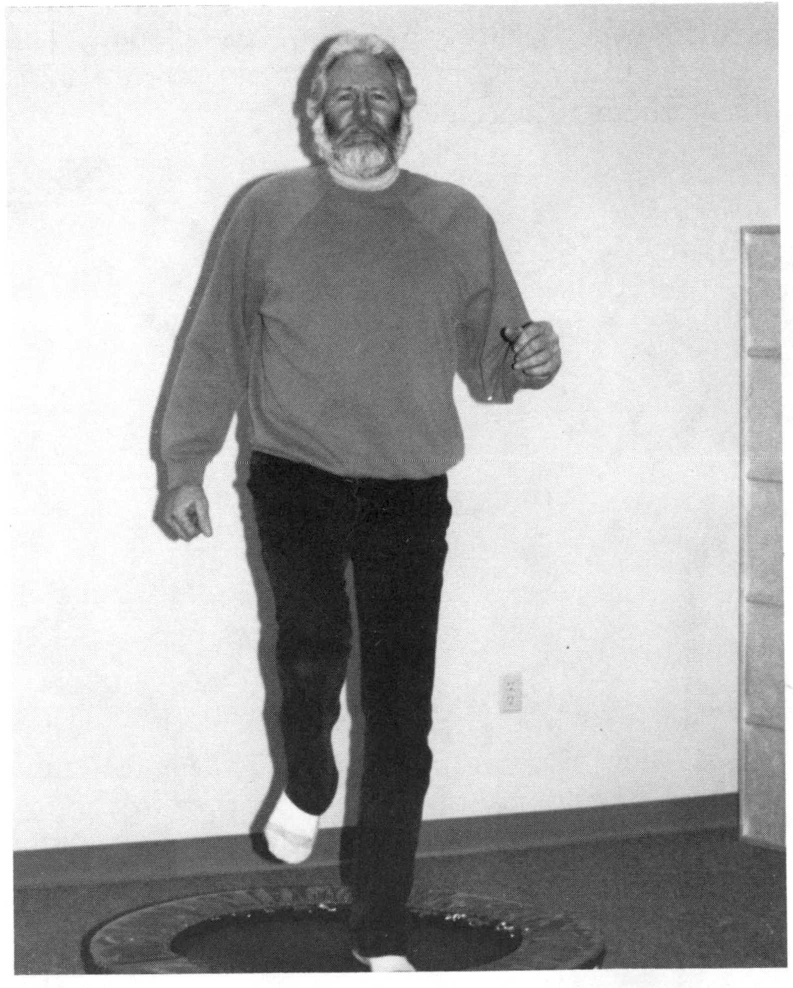

"REBOUNDING HAS HELPED KEEP MY LOWER BACK AND SKELETAL FRAME STRONG AND FLEXIBLE. JOGGING IN PLACE PUTS LESS STRAIN ON MY JOINTS WITH THE SAME BENEFITS AS ACTUAL JOGGING." HARVEY DAY

CHAPTER III

How Do You Move On It?

There are an endless number of fun ways you can move on the rebounder.

The message I want to convey first is <u>moderation</u>. Please avoid overdoing. This is a compact exercise. One of the popular reasons people offer for not using their rebounders is the fact that they get sore from working too hard for too long before their bodies became accustomed to the cellular exercise.

This is the most important chapter in this book. I'll explain <u>how</u> to use your rebounder so you do not get sore, hurt or bored. What you will get is the knowledge for starting a program for your likes and needs. You'll learn to walk before you run, bounce before you jump.

Simply speaking, there are four kinds of moves or bounces to use on the rebounder.

These are:

1. Health bounce
2. Strength bounce
3. Aerobic bounce
4. Sitting and optional bounces

The first three bounces can be utilized in most exercise sessions whether they are for aerobics or easy health maintenance. The fourth group of bounces includes those for specific training and therapy.

Now, the fun begins.

THE HEALTH BOUNCE

The health bounce means just that . . . bouncing for health.

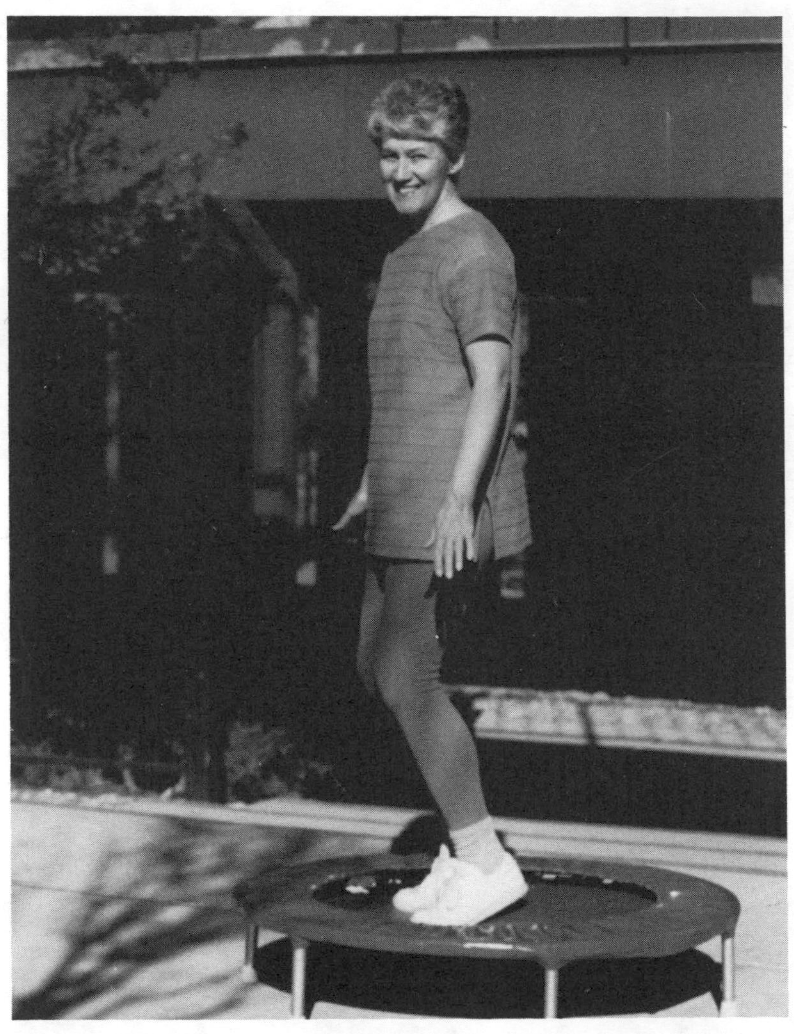

This is done by just <u>bouncing with feet on the mat</u>. Place your feet about 12 inches apart and shrug your shoulders or slightly lift your heels to get yourself bouncing. This gentle bouncing will strengthen every cell while flushing your lymphatics.

A couple of minutes of health bouncing is very effective for moving the lymph fluid, flushing toxins and waste products out of your body.

The lymphatic system is made up of a series of tubes that run throughout the body. Lymph is the clear fluid that bathes the cells, transports nutrients to the cells and takes waste products away from the cells. Lymph is moved like a hydraulic pressure system — not pumped by the heart. The lymph tubes are filled with one-way valves that only open up, or toward the center of the body. When pressure below the valve is greater than above, the valves are forced open, so the fluid can flow.

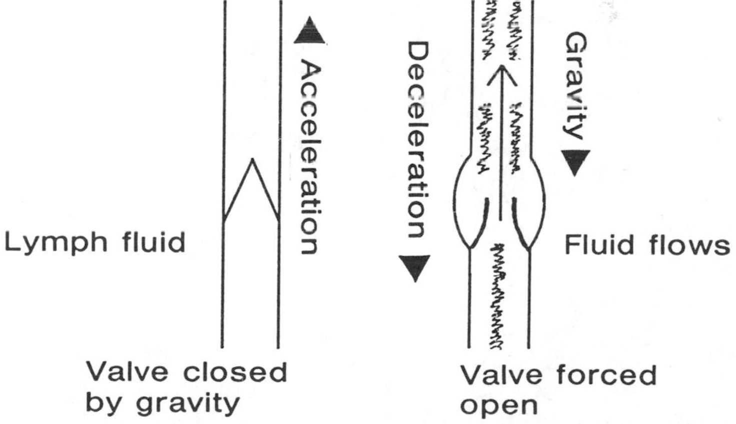

The rebounder can act as your lymph pump. At the bottom of the bounce, the gravitational pull closes the valves, but at the top of the bounce the pressure is decreased and the centrifugal force of your falling allows the lymph to flow up.

Because the lymph is flowing and waste is leaving, the body has a need for more white blood cells. In a few minutes of health bouncing, the white blood cells are increased as much as three fold.

Now, back to the health bounce. It can be an exercise by itself, done briefly 4-5 times a day. The health bounce is also a warm up and cool down bounce for aerobic or weight training sessions.

THE STRENGTH BOUNCE

The next move, the strength bounce, is done by actually jumping, so your feet leave the mat. The bottom line here is, if rebound exercise strengthens every cell of the body, then to concentrate on building strength, you just jump higher, increasing the G-force on each cell.

"MY REBOUND EXPERIENCE BEGAN IN 1981. IT HAS REMAINED MY MOST CONSTANT FORM OF EXERCISE THROUGH THE YEARS. I HAVE USED IT PRE, DURING AND POST NATALLY. THE REBOUNDER TAKES UP LITTLE SPACE IN A ROOM, CAN BE USED EVERY DAY OF THE YEAR, NO MATTER WHAT THE CONDITION OF THE WEATHER. REBOUNDING WAS A PERFECT EXERCISE FOR HELPING MY MOTHER-IN-LAW WHEN SHE WAS ILL. I SUPPLIED THE BOUNCE FOR HER IN A 'BUDDY-BOUNCE' SINCE SHE WAS QUITE WEAK WHEN WE BEGAN. EVENTUALLY SHE WAS ABLE TO BOUNCE ON HER OWN USING A STABILIZER BAR. (BECAUSE I WAS SO ENTHUSIASTIC ABOUT REBOUNDING, TWO FRIENDS BORROWED 2 OF MY REBOUNDERS AND WON'T PART WITH THEM.) WHEN I'M TIRED, ILL OR LAZY, I STILL MANAGE TO GET ON MY REBOUNDER FOR AT LEAST A LIGHT AND SHORT WORKOUT." PEGGY LANGENWALTER

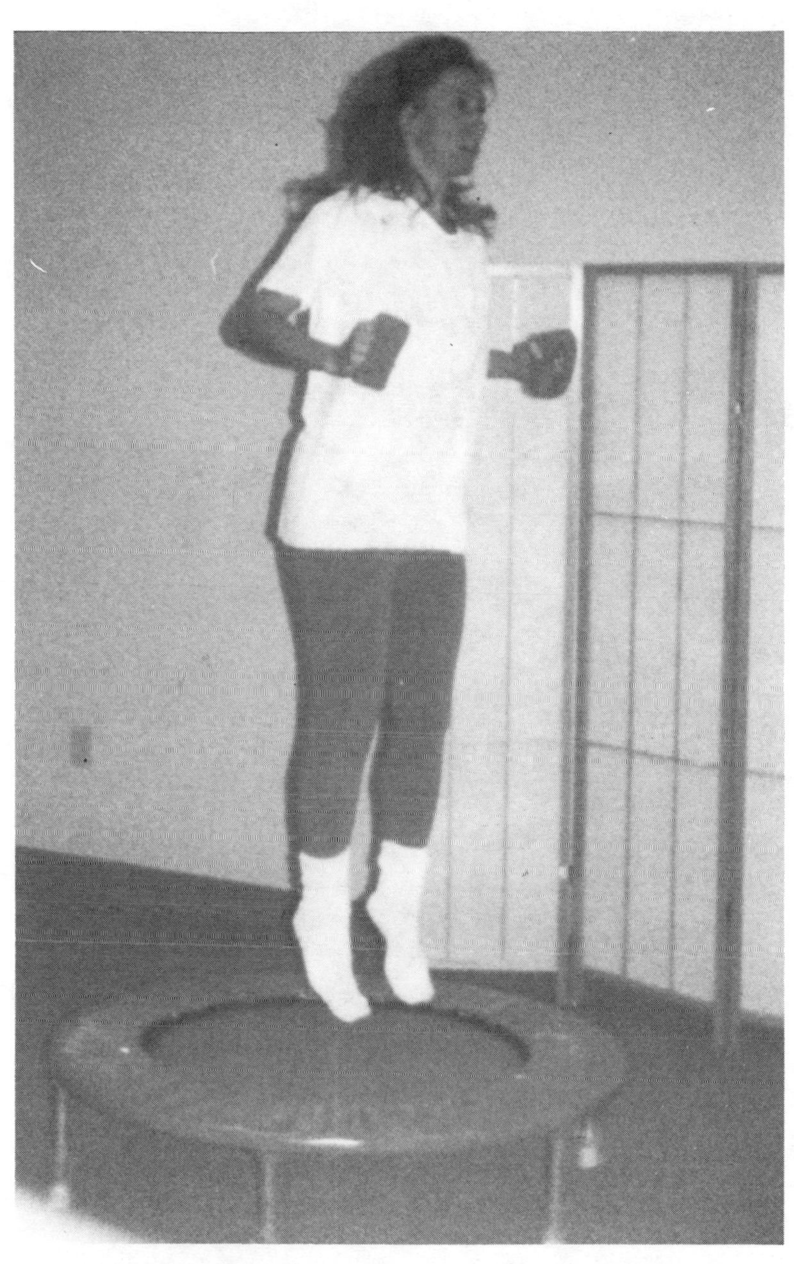

Peggy enjoying her strength bouncing.

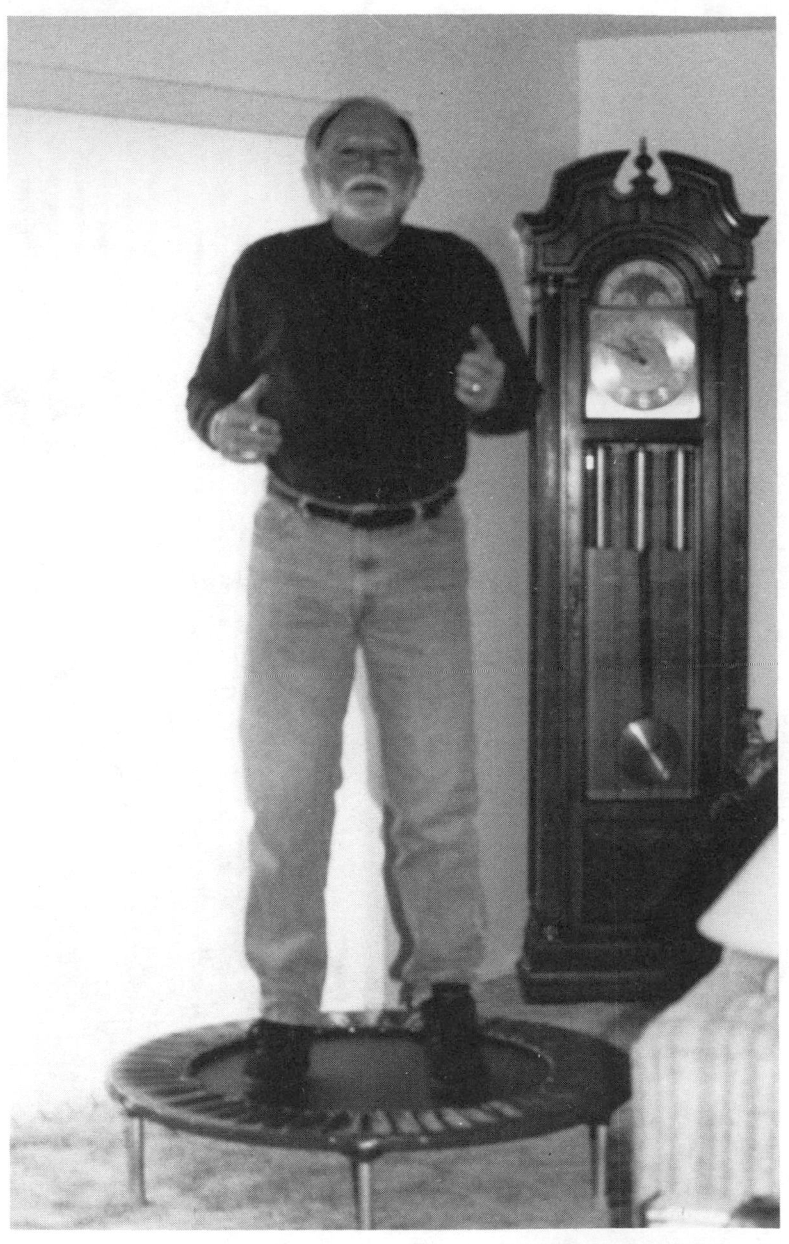

Michael Rivers bounces for strength.

THE AEROBIC BOUNCE

The aerobic bounce is versatile, creative, and fun. Aerobic bounces include jogging, sprinting, twists, jumping jacks and other fun moves. Because of the buoyancy and shock-resistant mat, you can really have fun with rebound aerobics.

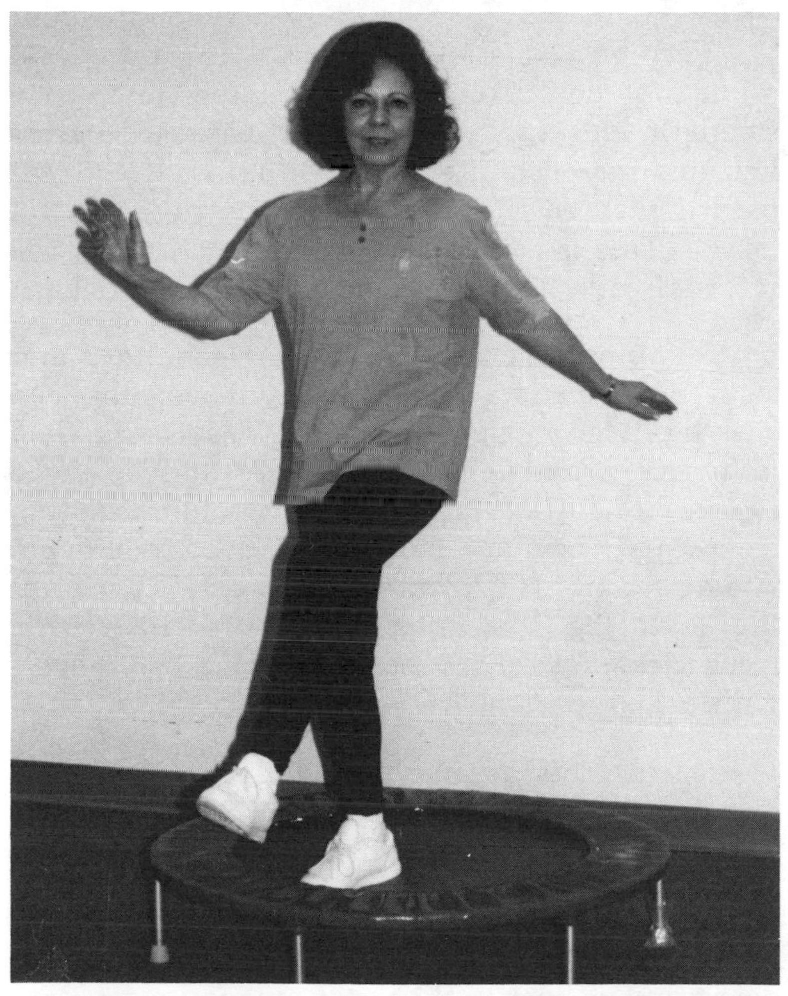

Theresa puts her best foot forward with the front kick.

"I PURCHASED MY REBOUNDER ABOUT 2 WEEKS AGO AND IT WAS THE BEST INVESTMENT I HAVE MADE IN A LONG TIME. I HAVE TAKEN AN AEROBICS CLASS BEFORE AND ALTHOUGH I ENJOYED THE EXERCISE, IT WAS VERY HARD ON MY FEET AMD MY CALVES. WITH THE REBOUNDER YOU GET THE EFFECTS OF AN AEROBIC EXERCISE BUT WITH NONE OF THE HARSH EFFECTS OF THE IMPACT. I FEEL GREAT!" THERESA HILDALGO

Turn on your upbeat music, warm up with a minute of health bounces, do a few jumps for strength, and start moving! Start easy, with arms low, and increase intensity gradually. If you feel pain anywhere, stop, rest, and continue a little later. (This is compact exercise that some of the internal cells may not be used to experiencing.)

Stepping side to side on the rebounder and swinging arms is a good start-up move. Proceed with light, easy jogging for about 30 seconds, then pull your arms up to heart level and do some twists, moving heels from side to side, twisting from waist down and moving upper body in opposite direction. Now, you can do a series of jumping jacks, leg lifts, knee to opposite elbow lifts, front kicks, fast short jumps, or other fun moves, with arms up at heart level.

During this aerobic period, a fast sprint for one minute is very effective for energizing the body. When changing motions, bouncing or jogging will help in the transition.

After 20 minutes of fun and exhilaration, slow down, and go back to the warm-up motions, bringing arms gradually back down to below heart level. When you have cooled down, finish with one minute of the health bounce to flushout the lactic acid and uric acid that might otherwise cause sore muscles.

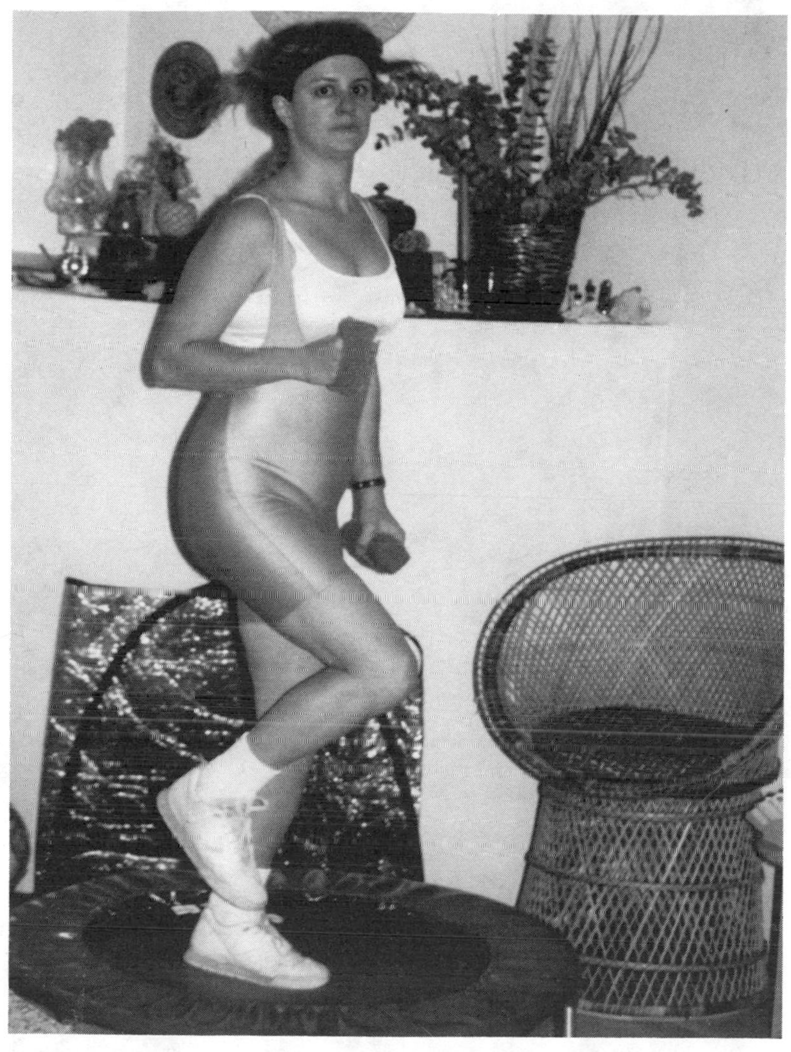

"I STARTED REBOUNDING IN AUGUST 1994. MY HUSBAND AND I LOVE IT! I DO 40 MINUTES EVERY DAY. IT GREATLY ENHANCES MY EQUESTRIAN ACTIVITIES AND I LOVE THE OVERALL CARDIOVASCULAR AND STRENGTH WORKOUT. IT MAKES ME FEEL VERY FIT!" JANISE BALDO-PULASKI

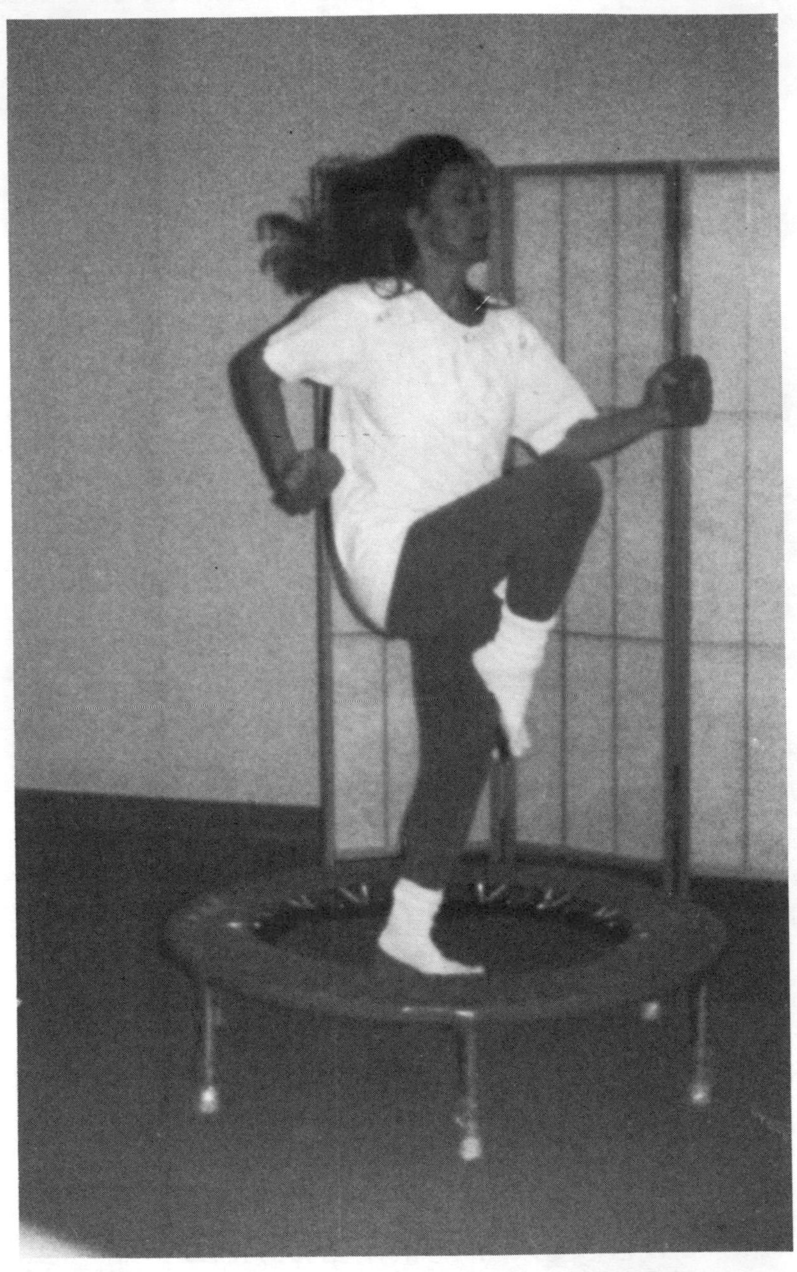

Here's Peggy high sprinting.

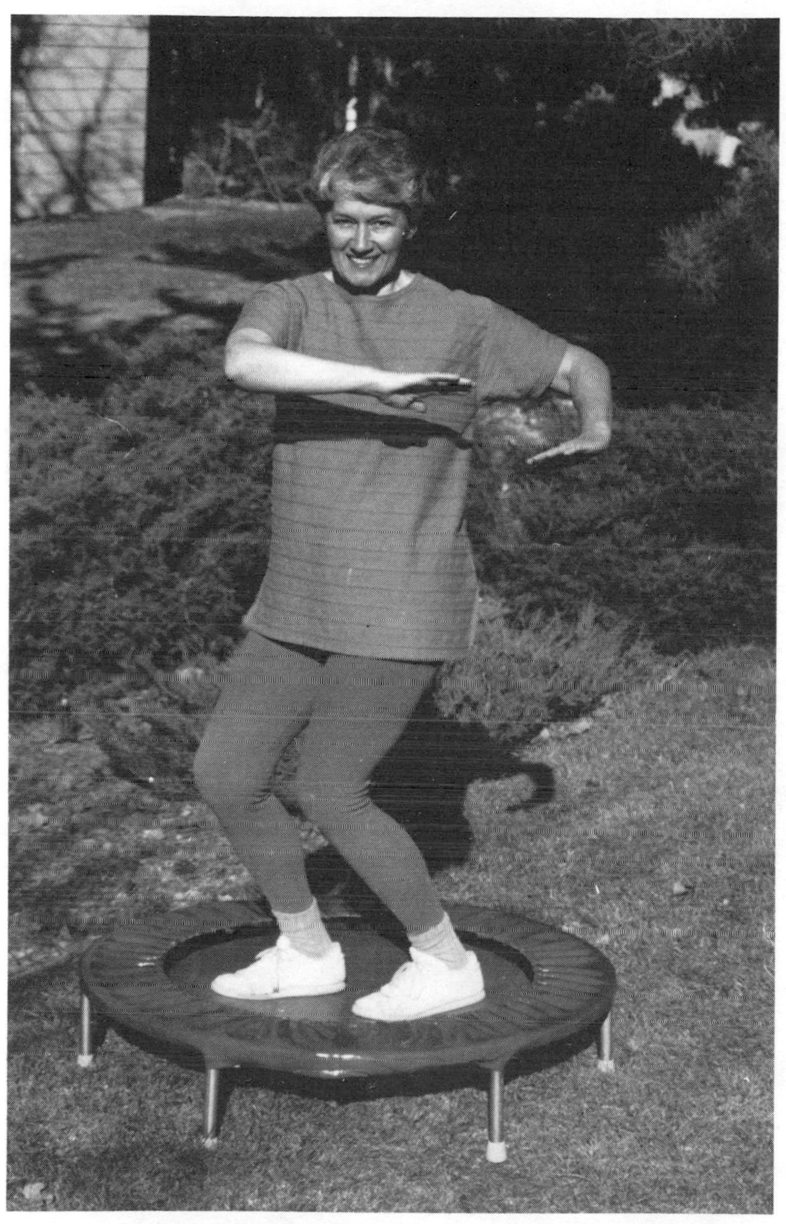

Linda demonstrates the "twist", her feet and hips turning to the right and her torso to the left.

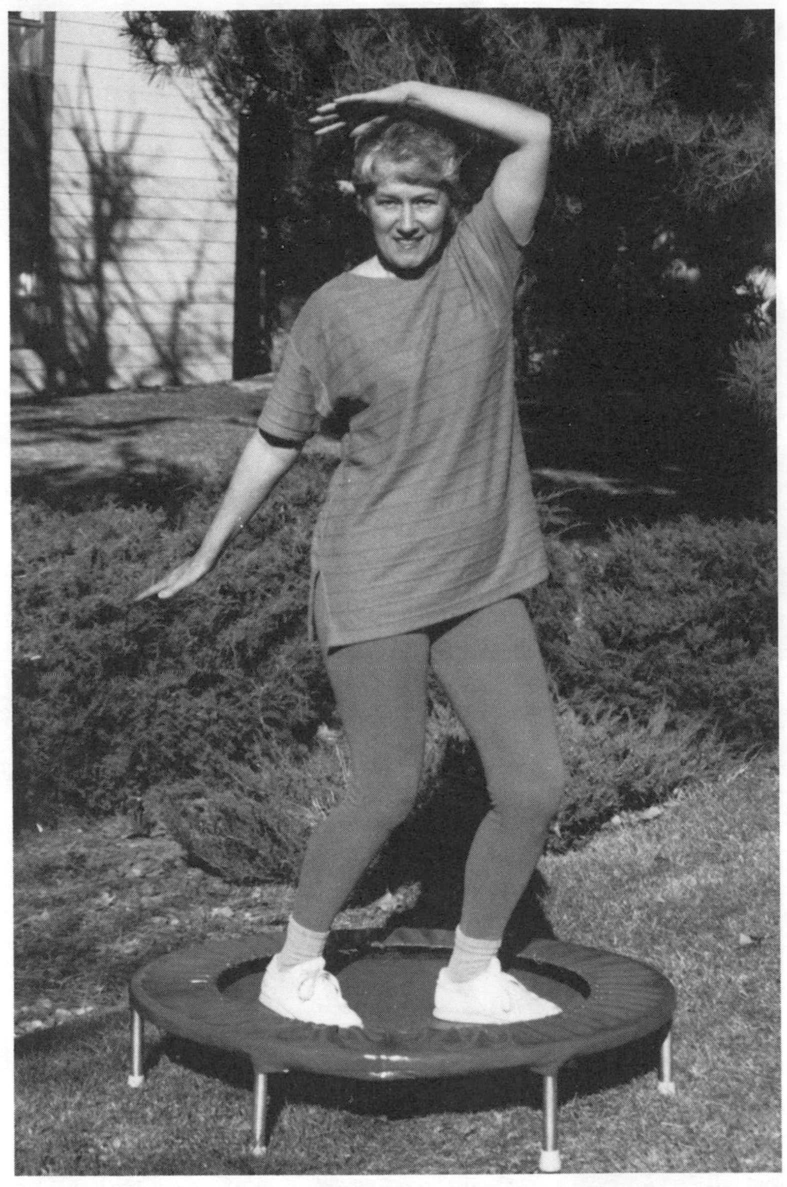

The "overhead twist".
The "twist" motions are excellent for toning stomach and waistline.

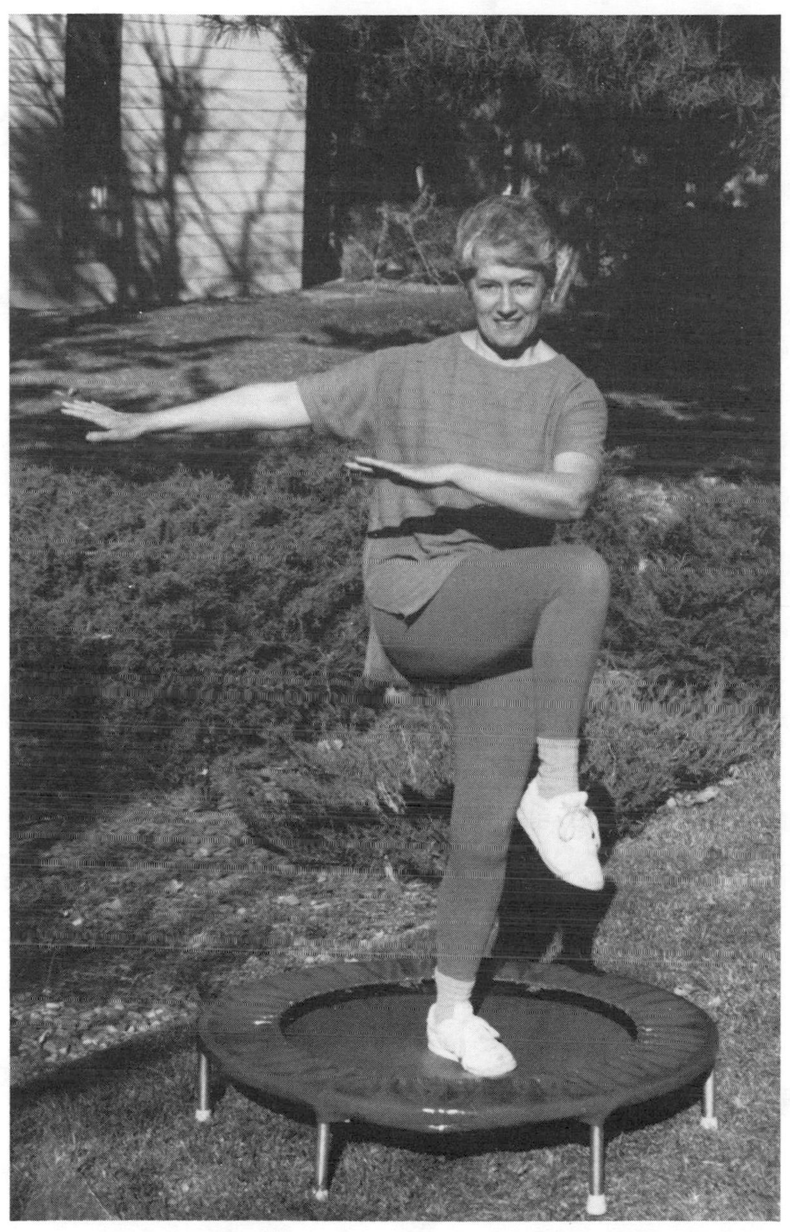

Cross crawls (right knee to left elbow and then reverse, left knee to right elbow).

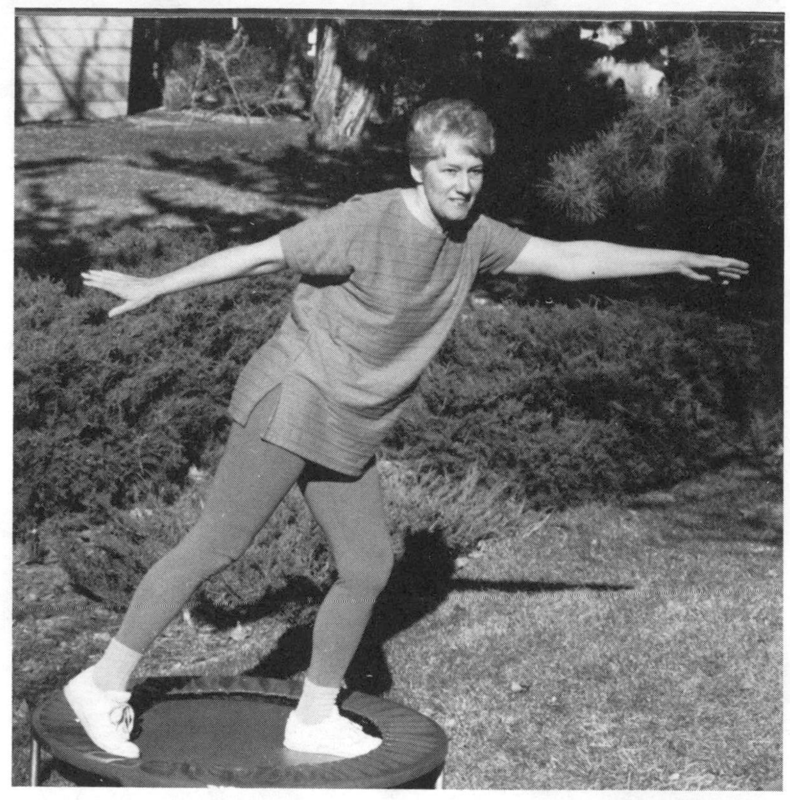

Back kick (really a stretch). Stand at the front of the mat and stretch right leg all the way to the back with left arm extended forward and then reverse with the left leg to the back and right arm forward. You'll feel as though you are pulling a rope in front of you. It is the pulling motion that helps you extend your arms.

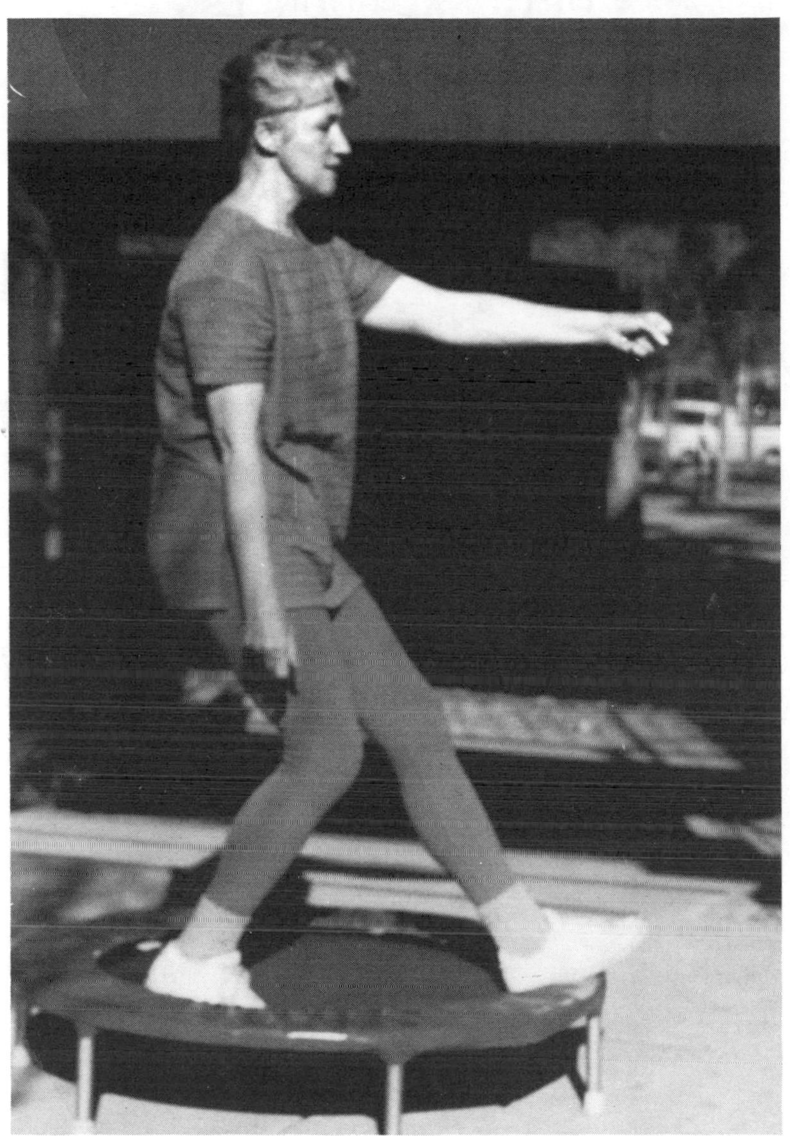

The shuffle is the partner to the back kick in that it is the reverse. Here Linda is kicking her feet forward in a shuffling motion. The arms are alternately stretching as if pulling on a rope.

OPTIONAL BOUNCES

The sitting and optional bounces prove that rebound exercise is truly for everyone. Since it is such a gentle and safe exercise, a person, who for some reason cannot stand on the rebounder, can sit on the mat and bounce, or let someone stand behind him or her and do the bouncing.

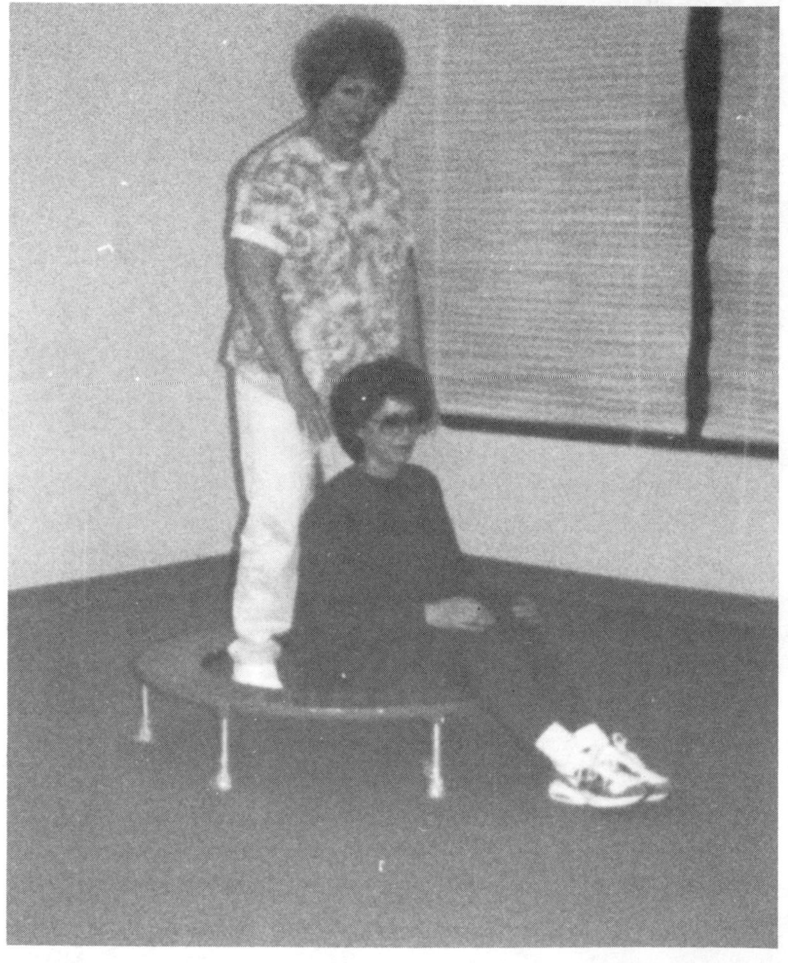

Linda and Rose are doing the “buddy bounce”.

This flushes the lymphatics and brings circulation and strength to the upper half of the body. After that session, the person moves to a chair, and puts his or her legs on the rebounder and lets someone else do the bouncing again. Now the entire body has been affected by rebound exercise.

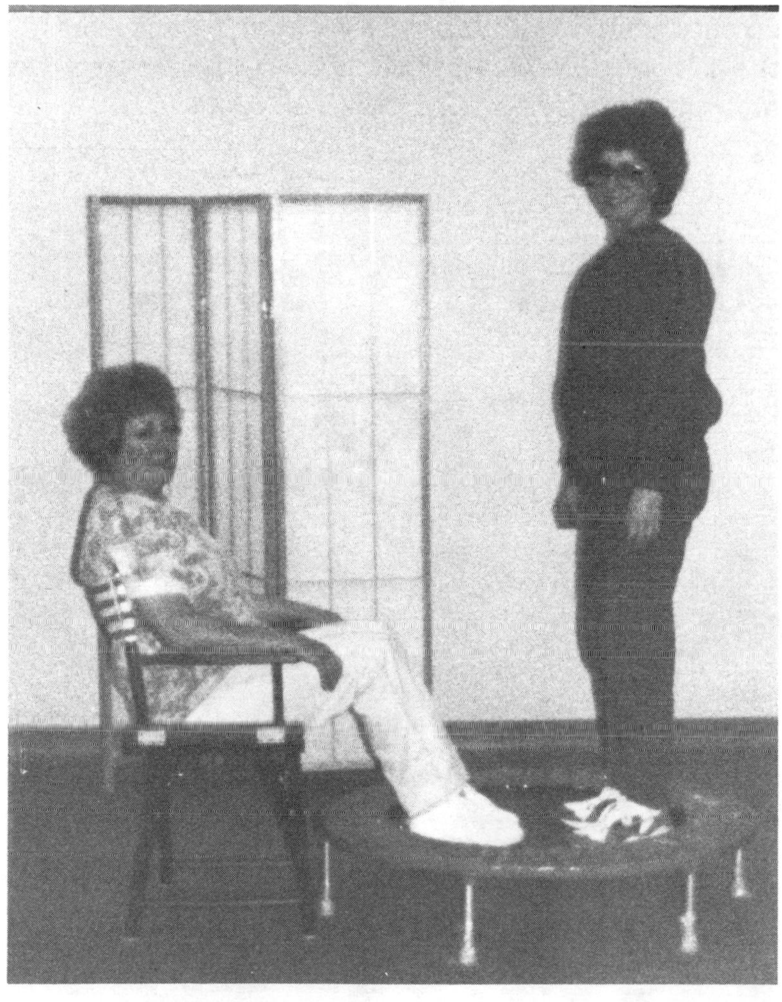

Linda receives the benefits of rebounding to her legs as Rose bounces.

As balance and strength are increased, the people who started with the sitting bounce can stand up and do the health bounce for 1-2 minutes, and work up to bouncing several times a day.

The sitting bounce can also be used to strengthen the abdominals, legs, and back. Sit on the rebounder, feet off the floor, and bounce by moving your arms in a circular motion.

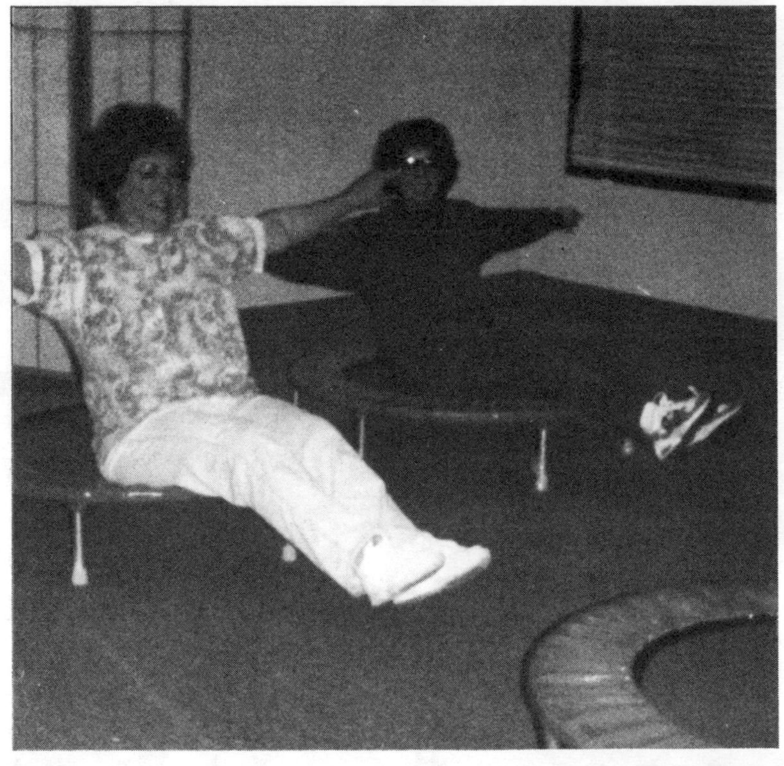

Linda and Rose are strengthening their abdominals.

As strength increases, you can pull your legs higher from the floor and lean back a little farther, while bouncing. The ultimate position for building strength is to bounce in a V position. This takes lengthy training, and should not be attempted by beginners.

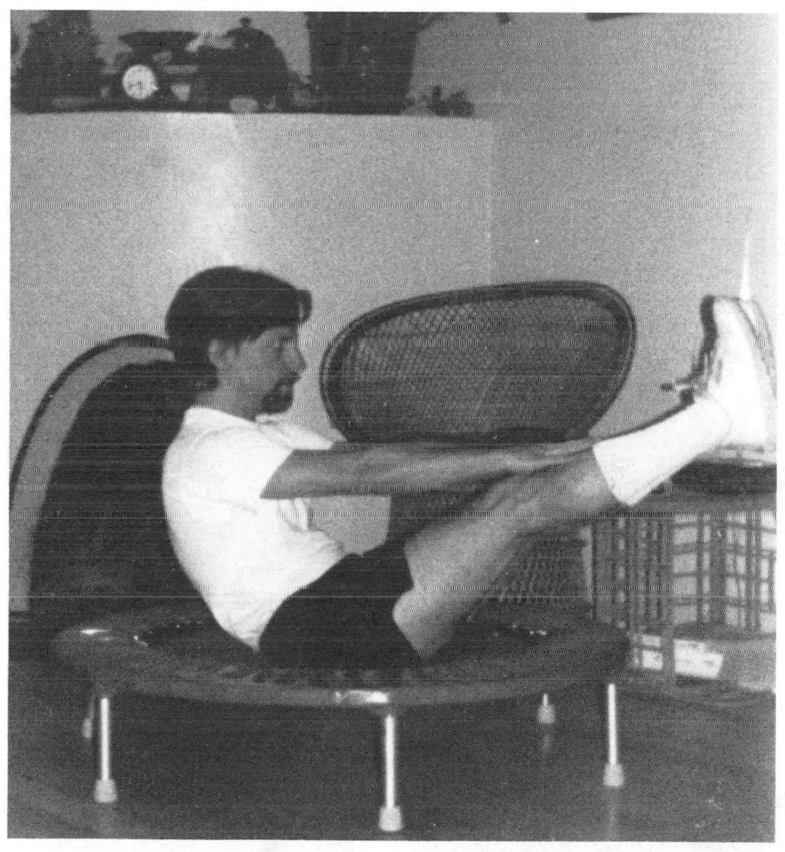

Paul demonstrates with ease the “V Bounce”.

7-MINUTE FITNESS

This is a wonderful exercise for busy people who want a quick, compact exercise that energizes, cleanses, and builds health and strength.

This routine should not be attempted by beginning rebound users or anyone with injuries who is still on a bouncing routine to rebuild health.

Be sure you can do 1-2 minutes of strength bouncing and a minute of jogging before attempting to put these moves together for this exercise. It's divided into two sessions of 3 1/2 minutes each. The first session is done early in your morning, and the other in the afternoon.

Each session of 3 1/2 minutes goes like this:

1. Health bounce for 30 seconds
2. Strength bounce for 1 minute
3. Fast sprint for 1 minute
4. Health bounce for 1 minute

Step 1 is your warm-up. In Step Two, you are telling your body you are really going to exercise. The one minute of fast sprinting is that heavy-duty exercise. Pace yourself throughout this minute so you increase it to full-speed-ahead during the last 15 seconds. Your intention is to give it all you've got, use up your ATP, and cause your mitochondria (your fuel-producing furnaces) to divide. This provides you with more ATP for vigorous exercise, but you can now cool down, equipped with more furnaces for producing energy for hours.

This routine may be repeated again in the afternoon for optimum energy all evening.

At night, while you sleep, your number of furnaces, goes back to normal, so in the morning, you can do the 3 1/2 minutes over again. It Works!

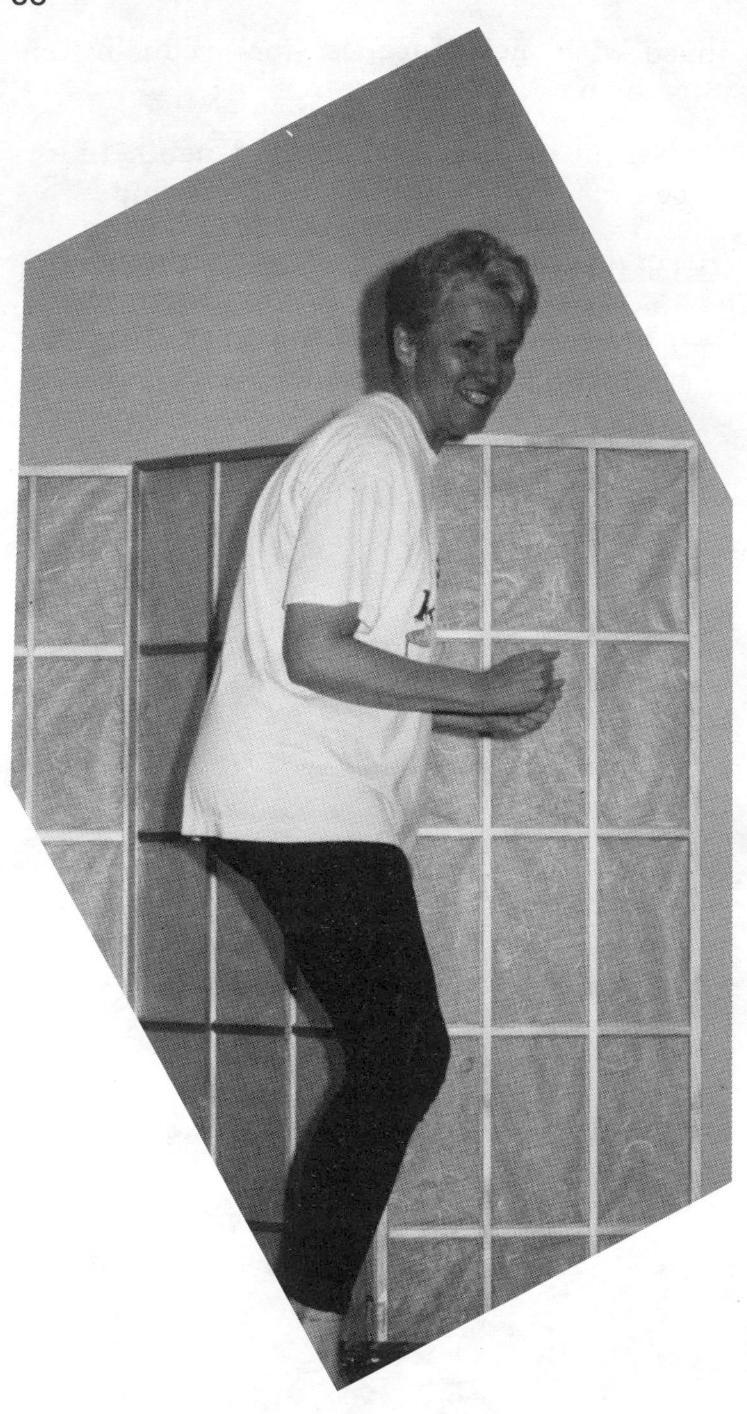

CHAPTER IV

Therapeutic Rebounding

In this chapter on therapeutic rebound moves, I will give a brief, simplified explanation of how rebound exercise can be very effective with a variety of physical conditions. With the understanding that every cell is strengthened and the lymph is moved effectively with this shock-free exercise, it is easy to see how this exercise benefits these specific conditions.

TRAPPED BLOOD PROTEINS

A very important aspect of rebound exercise is that it efficiently removes trapped blood proteins from around the cells where they hold fluid and can cause pain and disease. These blood proteins naturally get squeezed out of the capillary by cardiovascular pressure, but since there isn't enough pressure to force them back in, they collect around the cells, attracting fluid. Rebound exercise facilitates the movement of these trapped proteins into the lymphatic veins, excess fluid is removed, and the cells can receive oxygen again.

REBOUNDING AND ARTHRITIS

According to the Arthritis Foundation, "Arthritis is one of the supreme remaining mysteries of medicine." With a simple description of what arthritis is, I think you'll understand clearly how rebounding works so effectively in clearing up arthritic conditions, and you'll stop seeing arthritis as such a "mystery".

It is important to understand that the joints of the human body have no veins or lymphatic tubes. Circulation comes from movement. Movement squeezes old fluid out and new fluid in.

When a foreign invader enters a joint, lymphocytes, or white blood cells, come to the site to clean up the inflamed joint. They start eating, but because the joint isn't being moved, they cannot get out, so they overeat and spew out toxins that kill cells on the synovial lining of the joint. More lymphocytes come to the joint, eat, get trapped, spew toxins, and the situation gets worse. The white blood cells are just trying to do their job of cleaning up the dead cells, but because of lack of movement of the joint from pain, they just cannot get out.

The answer then, from a natural standpoint, seems to be to find a way to painlessly move that lymph fluid holding white blood cells full of waste, out of the inflamed joint, and ultimately, out of the body.

You got it. Gentle health bouncing flushes the lymph, the foreign body, the dead white blood cells and toxins out of the joint. New white blood cells come in, do their work, but this time, because of repeated bouncing sessions, they are flushed from the joint before they can spew out toxins. When the inflammation has subsided, gentle range of motion exercises re-establish movement to the joint.

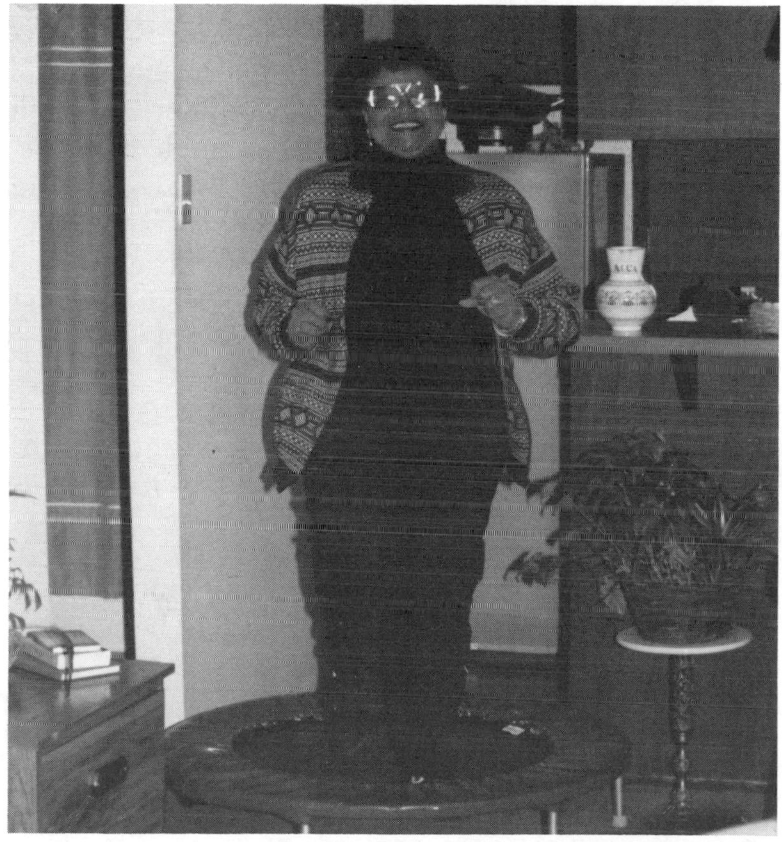

"REBOUNDING ENERGIZES MY BODY. IT ALSO RELAXES ME FROM HEAD TO TOE. I FEEL THE TENSION JUST FLOWING OUT OF ME. I ENJOY BOUNCING FACING THE FOUR DIRECTIONS ONE AT A TIME."
LUZ VALDES NORRIS

Regular health bouncing, light jogging, and working into a regular program of rebound exercise, will strengthen the tendons, ligaments, lining of the joints, and bones. Circulation is increased, more oxygen is carried to the cells, and the bones absorb more calcium. All this is done without pain, shock to the joints, or the inconvenience of leaving your home.

Start easily and slowly. Health bounce for 1-2 minutes every hour on the hour, or as many times a day as possible. Remember, if you feel pain while rebounding, stop, rest, and start again later. Some people start with 30 seconds of bouncing, and increase slowly to 1-2 minutes. Brief sessions, several times a day, are more therapeutic than 1 long session, because of the repeated movement of lymph and increased production of white blood cells.

Within 1-2 weeks you can lengthen your sessions, according to your pace of healing. Light jogging on the rebounder can be added, as well as other moves, as you are ready.

Start slowly and easily, and remember to be steady with your bouncing, and you will be pleased with the progress, with no side effects!

OSTEOPOROSIS

With the rising incidence of osteoporosis, this condition has become a household word. Many factors contribute to this malady, but rebound exercise is whole-body, cellular exercise, and can be very effective in preventing the devastating effects of osteoporosis.

It is a well-known fact that bones become stronger when stressed. Bone cells deposit more minerals in bone tissue with the greatest amount of stress, and remove minerals from bones with the least amount of stress. From this, you can see that bones become stronger when stressed by exercise, and weaker without it. In just 14 days, the astronauts who went to the moon, lost 15% of their bone density because there was no gravitational pull to positively stress their bones.

Osteoporosis occurs when there is more absorption of minerals from the cells than the deposition of minerals to the cells. Rebound exercise provides an avenue for stressing the bones to become dense and strong. The acceleration and deceleration, combined with the increased pull of gravity, stresses the bone cells so more mineral deposition takes place.

Brief periods of health bouncing and jogging is an excellent way to build bone density to prevent this dreaded disease. If osteoporosis is already present, then beginning a rebounding program and consuming a healthy, whole foods diet with fresh flax seed oil added will give you very basic building blocks for strong bones.

Start slowly and build up, but be consistent!

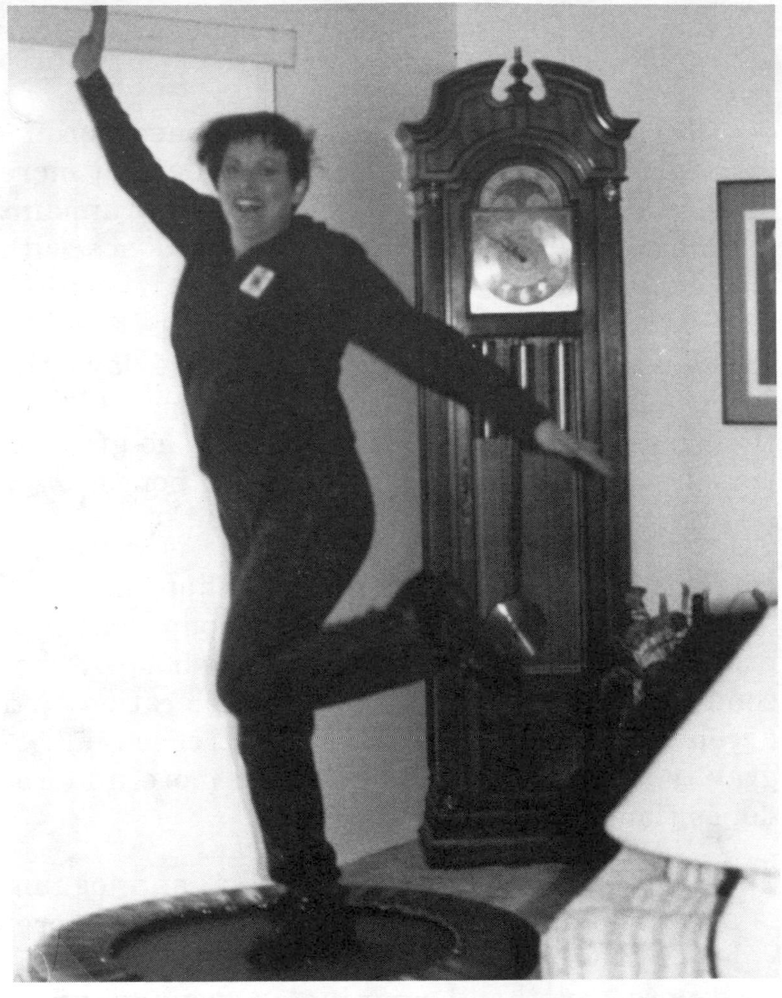

"I FEEL SO FREE AND OPEN LIKE FLOATING ON A CLOUD. I ALSO GET STRENGTH IN MY LEGS AFTER BOUNCING. I'VE HAD BOTH ANKLES BROKEN AND WHEN THEY ACHE, I REBOUND TO TAKE THE PAIN AWAY." YVONNE LEGENDARY RIVERS

VARICOSE VEINS

When the walls of the veins are too weak to support the blood moving toward the heart, the veins widen and pooling ofthe blood occurs, causing more stretching.

Rebound exercise strengthens the cells of the veins, building strength in the veins to support proper blood flow. With health bouncing several times a day, circulation is improved, and the injured veins heal. Little spider veins disappear, usually within a few weeks and continued healing takes place with consistent daily health bouncing, up to 5 minutes, 4-5 times a day.

INCONTINENCE/BLADDER CONTROL

This is a vastly growing problem, with adult diapers being a billion dollar industry. More and more seniors are losing the ability to control their urinary water loss. However, this problem is quite prevalent among people who are much younger, some in their late 20's or early 30's. No matter what the age, the answer lies in strengthening the sphincter muscles that control the flow of urine from the bladder.

Bouncing on a rebounder may not, at first, sound too appealing to someone who has a bladder control problem, but it is just what is needed. Since rebound exercise is cellular, it strengthens the cells of the sphincter muscles, building increased control of the bladder within about 2 weeks.

Begin exercising with short periods of health bouncing, several times a day, every day. Stop and use the bathroom when needed, and get back on your rebounder.

As you build strength in your muscles, you will be able to exercise with less and less trips to the bathroom. Within a few weeks to a few months, depending on your rebounding program, you can resume normal activities without the nagging fear of incontinence.

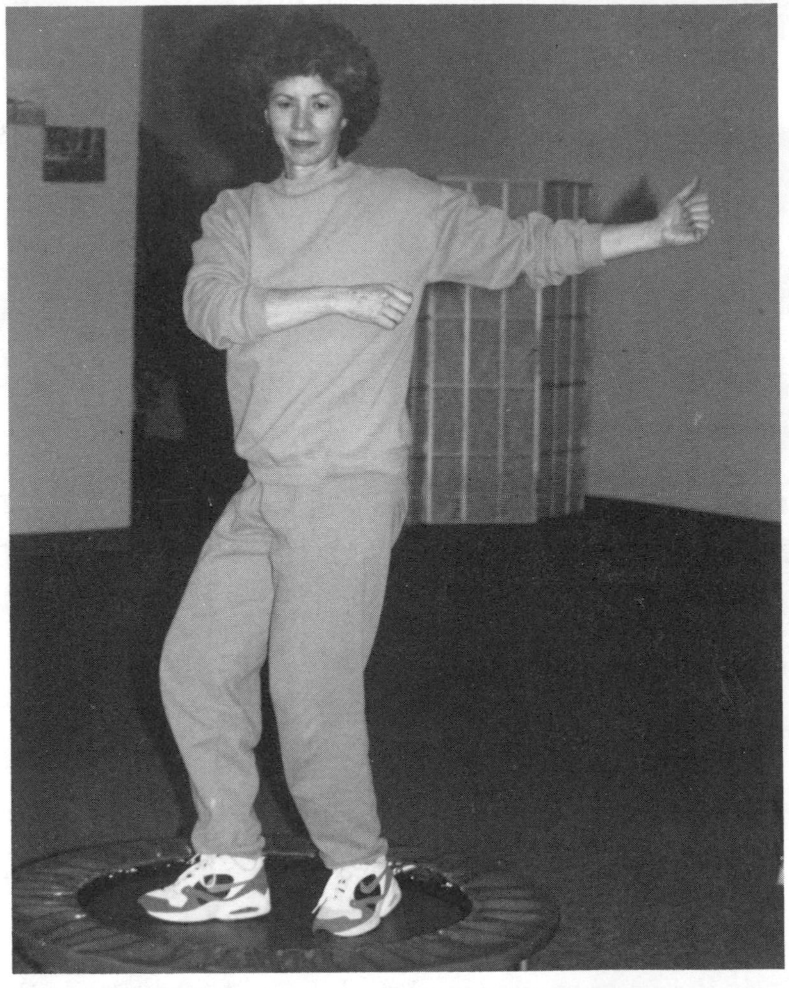

"AFTER INCONTINENCE PROBLEMS, I FOUND OUT ABOUT THE REBOUNDER AND AFTER ABOUT 1 1/2 MONTHS MY PROBLEM HAS DIMINISHED GREATLY; IN ADDITION, I HAVE MORE ENERGY AND MY BODY SEEMS TO BE FIRMER." ROSE ARNELL

A good routine would be 1-2 minutes of health bouncing 4-5 times a day for the first week. The second week, increase to 3 minutes each time, and the third week increase to 5 minutes, 4-5 times a day. Add light jogging if you like. Have fun, think health and healing. It's taking place as you bounce!

WEIGHT LOSS

Rebound exercise, accompanied with a healthy diet of whole grains, fresh fruits and vegetables, the elimination of margarines and other hydrogenated fats, and the addition of a healthy oil like fresh flax oil, makes the weight loss process natural and hassle-free.

Regular, repeated sessions of rebound exercise will build stronger cell walls for better tone and less fat storage. With rebound exercise, inches will be lost where needed, and gained where desired.

You are able to burn more calories per hour with rebounding than with regular exercise and with 87% less shock, less effort, and more safety. The number of calories burned per hour by a 154 pound person are:

1440 Sprinting on rebounder
750 Regular running
600 Rebound jogging
420 Bicycling at 10 MPH
150 Health bouncing
150 Indoor walking

During the health bounce, you are flushing the lymphatics, adding strength to every cell and improving metabolism, circulation, vision and hearing, plus many other benefits, making this exercise more efficient than regular walking.

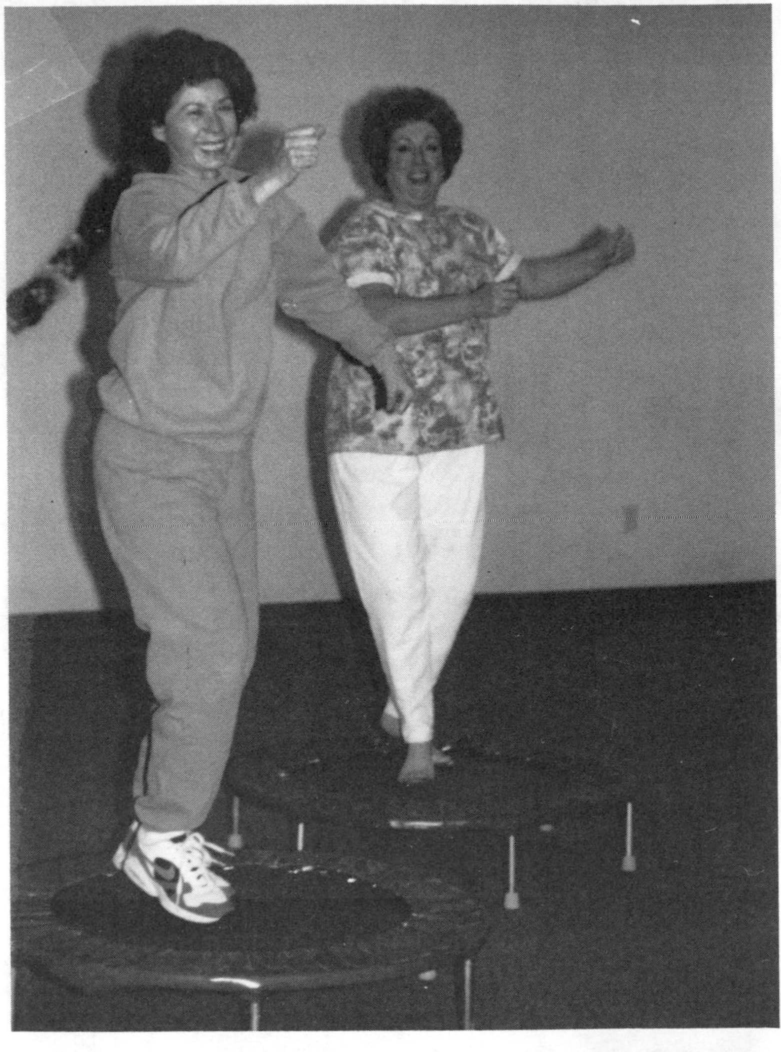

Linda and Rose move to the music during their rebounding aerobics class.

Here's another plus for rebound running, jogging, or other aerobic moves. You get your heart rate up with less effort because of your buoyancy combined with acceleration and deceleration This also makes it easier to maintain the aerobic state, so exercise becomes fun! Turn on upbeat music and jog, twist, run, and jump through several songs. Vary your motions so you don't get bored, and time will fly.

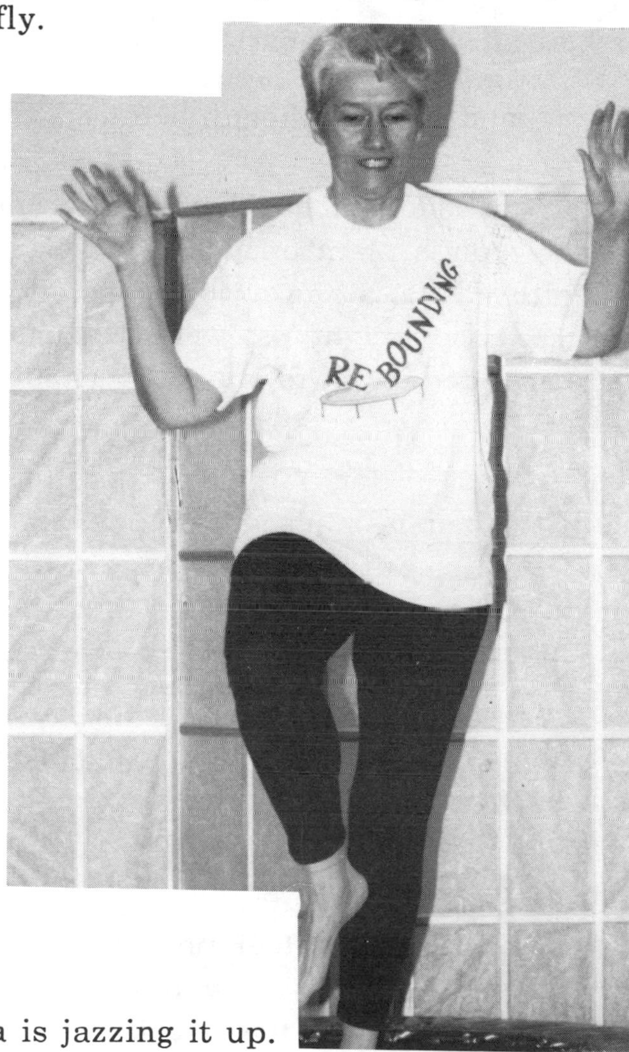

Linda is jazzing it up.

A sample program might include:

- 2-3 minutes of health bouncing first thing in the morning.
- Mid-morning aerobic session, starting easy and working up to 20-40 minutes.
- Health bounce for 3 minutes, 30 minutes before meals.
- Late afternoon and early evening sessions of 1 minute health bounce, 1 minute jogging, and 1 minute health bounce.

When you build total health with diet, complete digestion through plant enzymes and cleansing with healthy flora, along with consistent daily rebound exercise, weight loss will occur naturally, almost as a side benefit to your new vitality and joyful life.

The biggest obstacle in weight loss for most people is the emphasis placed on time. You want instant results, but you didn't get this way overnight, although it may seem that you did. Be patient and consistent.

Be sure to take body measurements as well as weight before starting a rebounding program. Redistribution takes place, and that's exciting and encouraging.

Progress is charted individually, but on the whole, you can expect to feel more energetic and notice subtle differences as well as weight loss suited to you during the first week. During the second week, you should really see changes. After four weeks, you can experience weight and inches lost, more vitality, strength, better muscle tone, sleeping better and more.

If you don't like, or don't feel able to do aerobic exercises, then easy bouncing in short repeated sessions and 30 minutes before each meal can work very well for you, too, to build health and tone throughout the body, while appeasing the appetite.

Be consistent and support your rebounding program with nutritious sugar-free, low fat, nutrient dense foods and start building a glowing healthier you.

CANCER

The human body was created by God with the ability to heal itself of serious illness, as well as colds and flu, by way of a strong, healthy immune system. The power of rebound exercise to stimulate the immune system is virtually unknown by the majority of people, yet this simple easy exercise has helped relieve many people of cancerous conditions.

Because of its boost to the immune system and ability to completely flush the lymphatics in 2 minutes, rebound exercise, in my opinion, should not be overlooked where cancer is concerned. I have seen tumors leave clients who health bounced 2-3 minutes of every waking hour consistently, followed a healthy diet for cleansing and healing, and supported this with a strong belief in getting well.

During the health bounce, the toxins and wastes are being removed, so a new supply of white blood cells is called in, triple in number. In one hour the WBC count is back to normal, so health bouncing every waking hour keeps the WBC's optimum in the body and the lymph moving.

An optimum diet is essential to healing, as is the program you play in your mind. As described in Chapter IX, rebounding lowers the brain waves, making your mind very programmable. During every health bounce session every hour, the cancer patient would do well to create health and joy in his/her mind, and extend it to the body through that cellular mind-body connection.

Getting well does not have to be complicated and expensive, or debilitating. Cleanse out the toxins, add a healthy diet, enzymes with and between meals, clean, filtered water, rebound every hour, and believe in wellness!

VISION

Improved vision can be achieved in a relatively short period of time when eye exercises are done consistently on the rebounder. The lens of the eye changes shape because of lack of exercise, negatively affecting your vision. When glasses are added there is no stimulus for the lens to get stronger. With more lack of exercise to the cells of the lens, the best you can hope for is a prescription for stronger glasses, one after the other.

Rebound exercise, remember stimulates every cell to get strong. By doing eye exercises while health bouncing, you stimulate the lens of the eye to come back to its original shape, correcting your vision.

Position your rebounder about two feet from a window. Find a point on the window you can use for a focal point, or place something like a sticker on the window. Position your rebounder so your focus of the object is sharp. Now look out the window and find an object that you can see at a distance (street sign, pole, tree, branch). Begin health bouncing and focus on the near object, then far, then near, and back and forth. You are exercising the lens while stimulating it to get stronger. Remove your glasses or contact lenses. Repeat this exercise as many times a day as you can. The more frequently you practice this, the sooner you will see results. Done consistently, you can experience 20-50% improvement in the first three weeks. It's possible to correct your vision by consistently exercising the eyes in this manner two times a day for approximately six months.

The vision improvements need to be supported by continued exercise on the rebounder of course. This also helps protect against cataracts and other eye disorders.

SAGGING, BAGGING AND WRINKLING

The concept of aging, wrinkling, and shrinking like a prune, inside and outside, seems to be accepted in mostpeople's minds as an inevitable fact of life. The pull of gravity plays a natural role in this process as we move about daily, and we have to oppose gravity with every move. Cell walls also become weakened from lack of exercise, stress, free-radicals and chemicals.

What seems like a losing battle becomes the opposite with rebound exercise, accompanied with an optimum diet. Since rebound exercise strengthens and tones every single cell of the entire body, the skin and internal organs are stimulated to become stronger and firmer. With regular rebounding, the skin will become more subtle with fewer wrinkles. Badly wrinkled skin takes on firmer tone and can appear less wrinkled. Since rebound exercise does not tear down tissue from shock or exertion, but instead brings oxygen, nutrients, and increased circulation to cells, accompanied with the acceleration, deceleration, and gravity, it rebuilds the cells. It should be very apparent to you by now that rebound exercise will not cause sagging breasts, but on the contrary, build firmer, fuller breasts as collagen is rebuilt.

By this same re-building process, prolapsed organs are toned and rebuilt as they regain their normal strength.

Gain healthy glowing skin and internal tone while you strengthen your immune system and exercise your heart without expensive creams, oils, and facials. You get a facial and a massage every time you rebound!

A WORD TO HEALTH PRACTITIONERS

This wonderful cellular exercise supports and compliments other tools for natural healing marvelously. The toxins released during a massage can be effectively flushed out of the body by health bouncing. Acupuncture, chiropractic, and so much more can be supported by rebound exercise. Rebounding is the most effective way to move lymph and strengthen the entire body, leading to homeostasis, which makes it so compatible with other natural avenues for healing.

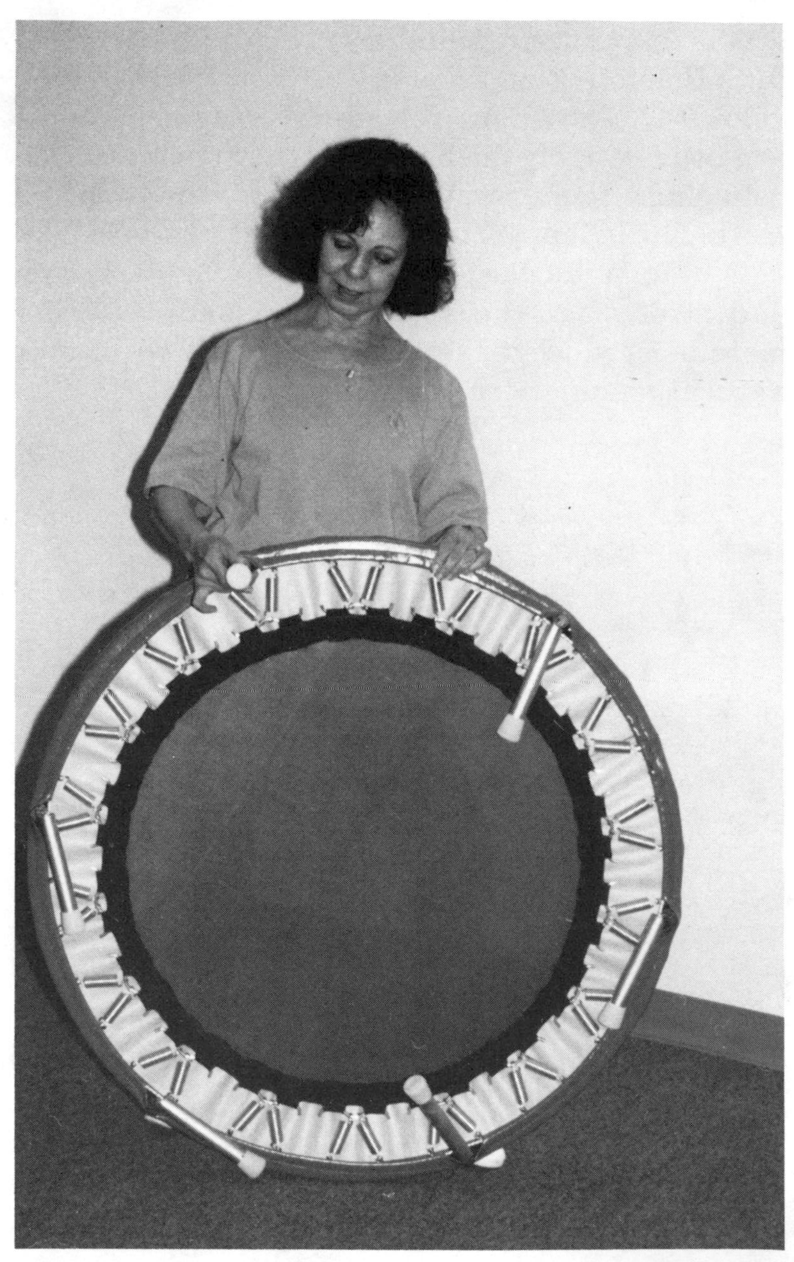

CHAPTER V

Weight Training and Athletics

Because rebound exercise is a cellular exercise, it can improve the efficiency of weight training and the skill and accuracy of a variety of sports. Weight training becomes more efficient while rebounding because of the buoyancy combined with the increased work load. Simply stated, as you jump on the rebounder and sink down into the mat, you create a force as if your body weighed twice what it does, or two G's (gravitational force). If you hold hand weights or use leg weights, the force is even greater, but because of the springing up and down, you don't feel the entire weight force. Your body reacts to it, stimulating muscles to become stronger even faster. Repeat this increased stress over and over, and you build strength.

Rebound exercise combined with circuit training has shown greater fat metabolism, greater muscle definition, and improved strength and endurance. In circuit weight training, instead of resting between exercise stations, rebound jogging is done.

A study incorporating 30 seconds of running or jogging on a rebounder between exercise stations shows that in only 12 weeks, strength was increased 26%, endurance improved by 17% and body fat percentages were reduced to 10.97%-17.1%.

Rebounding combined with weight training adds aerobic exercise to the anaerobics of body-building. You can achieve greater cardiovascular benefits, and rapid removal of lactic acid and waste products.

Rebound exercise improves balance, coordination, kinesthetic awareness, timing, and rhythm as it increases strength and endurance which makes it the ideal exercise for all sports enthusiasts. To really fine-tune your moves used in your particular sport, practice individual arm or leg moves while gently bouncing.

CHAPTER VI

Rebounding In The Work Place

The work place is one of the most important places for the rebound exercise. In the first place people spend a good percentage of their day there. In the second place, they are expected to perform with efficiency, accuracy, and show up in good health day after day with few days off for illness or rest. Doesn't this sound like a place where the life-giving benefits of rebound exercise would be helpful to employer and employee alike?

Since this exercise is cellular, it certainly will stimulate brain cells, increasing oxygen to the brain so employees can think more clearly. It provides increased stamina and greater immunity for employees, lowering the incidence of sickness, which brings health care costs down. Production can be greatly increased if employees are provided the opportunity to rebound for short periods several times throughout the day. Rebounding reduces stress, adds more accuracy, as well as efficiency, no matter what the type of job being done.

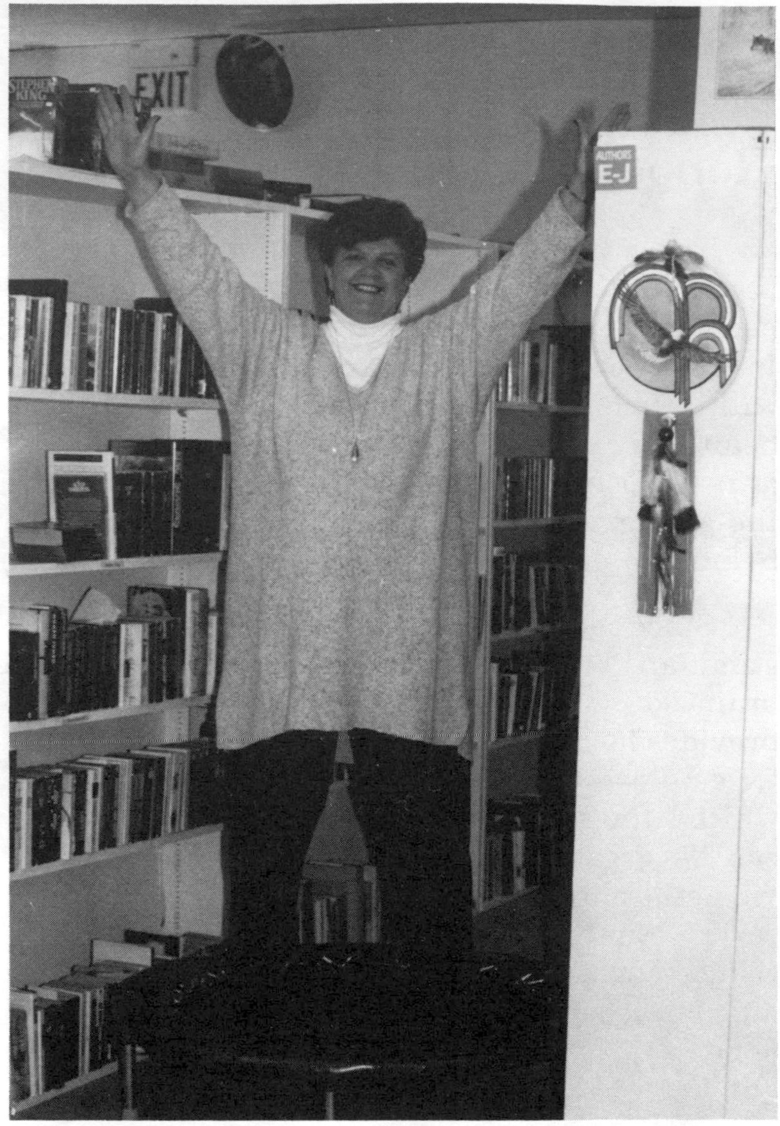

"AS AN OWNER OF A RETAIL BOOK STORE, I AM ON MY FEET SEVEN DAYS A WEEK. I ALWAYS HAD PAIN IN MY LEGS AND FEET THAT I LIVED WITH DAILY. REBOUNDING AT WORK HAS CHANGED ALL THAT. KEEPING A REBOUNDER IN OUR LECTURE ROOM ALLOWS ME TO BOUNCE TO RELIEVE THE STRESS ON MY FEET AND LEGS AND HELPS ME TO GET THROUGH THE DAY WITH MORE ENERGY AND LESS PAIN." SANDRA MCGILL

One major advantage of having rebounders in the work place involves the electro-magnetic waves streaming from computers all day long. This energy can shift your own electrical charge so you feel short-circuited and drained of energy. A few short minutes of rebounding reconnects that circuit, re-establishing your charge so you are grounded again, ready to work with precision.

Rebounders belong in all areas of the work place - the office, break room, and exercise room, if there is one. A business owner in California, started with one rebounder for himself, then bought 6 units for his employees. When he noticed positive results from his employees, he purchased 40 more rebounders. What he noticed was a marked reduction in stress reactions, increased production, more physical capabilities, uplifted spirits, reduction in absenteeism, and employees looked and acted healthier and more cheerful.

Rebound exercise can be adapted to any work place, large or small. Units spaced throughout a large office gives employees a chance to health bounce 1-2 minutes four or five times throughout the day, with longer bouncing at break-times. This brings relaxation, creativity, and clear thinking with vibrant energy, helping people enjoy their jobs.

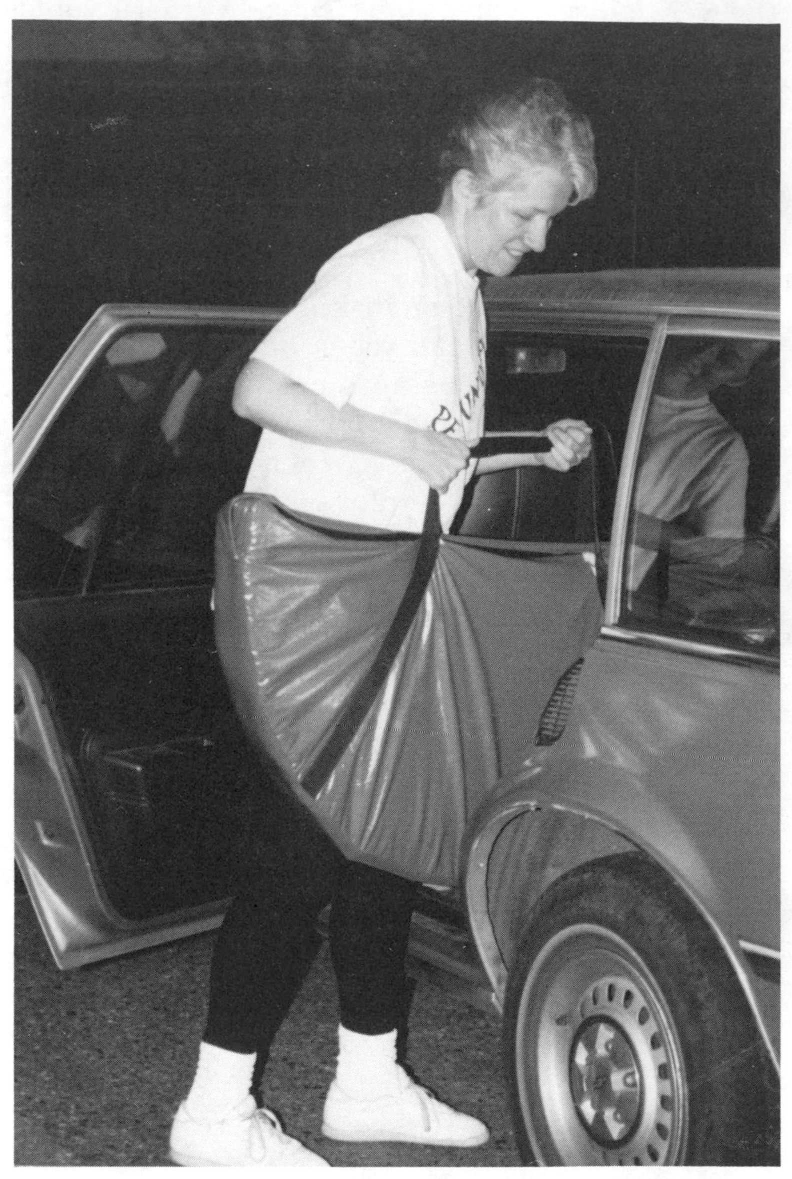

CHAPTER VII

Rebounding and Education

This cellular exercise that stimulates every cell of the brain certainly can be very effective in the education process. At least 30 chemicals in the cerebral-spinal fluid bathe the brain continuously. Rebound exercise stimulates the circulation of these fluids, improving mental activity.

At the bottom of the bounce, each brain cell is stimulated, making this an activity that improves memory, stimulates the thought process, and activates mental communication to each cell of the body. The brain waves are slowed to the alpha level. This is the frequency on which a child's brain operates, which is a very programmable state, where memory is enhanced and learning takes place. Health bouncing can, then, be beneficial in the education process of anyone. There are an unlimited number of ways for rebound education to be used.

Rebound education has been very effective in the classroom for many years. Students with learning difficulties benefit with improved eye-hand coordination and reading ability. Students can speed up the memorization of times tables or other rote material by repeating it while health bouncing. Balance and coordination are also improved.

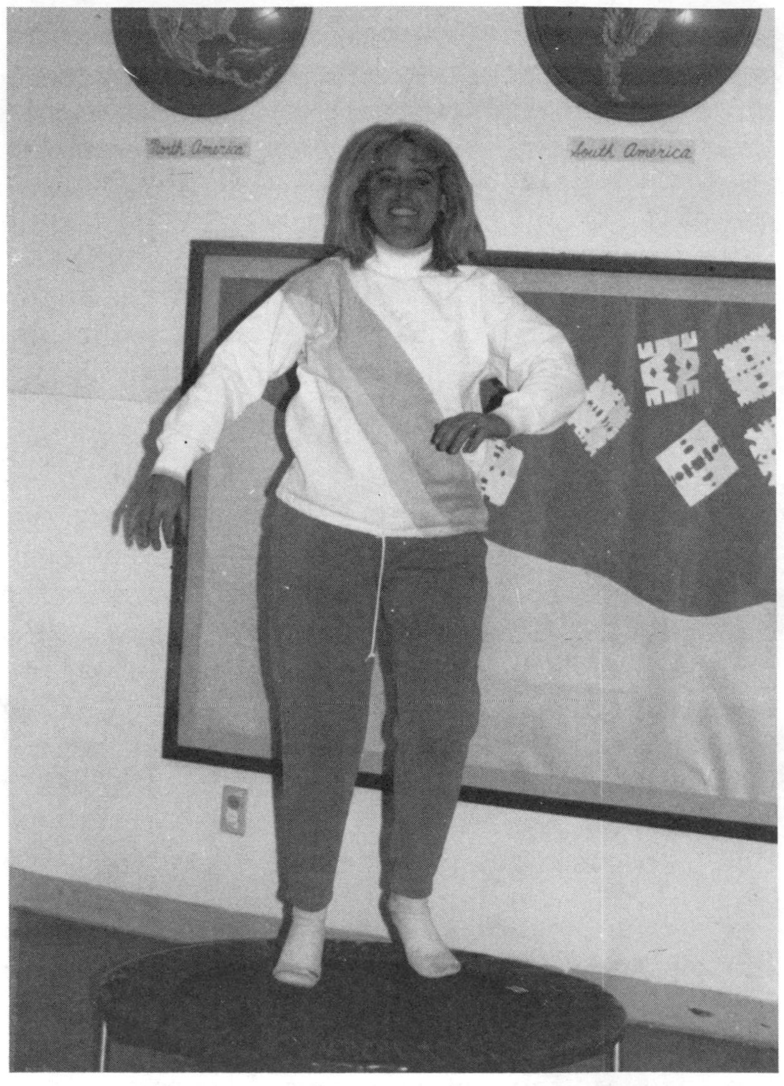

"I PUT THE REBOUNDER IN FRONT OF THE TV AND BEGAN BOUNCING AND BOUNCING AND IN NO TIME I WAS HUFFING AND PUFFING AS WELL AS SWEATING. I BEGAN TO HAVE A HAPPIER ATTITUDE AND MY SELF ESTEEM BECAME ENHANCED FROM THE DAILY JUMPING. I SINCERELY LOOK FORWARD TO JUMPING THE FOLLOWING DAY; IT DOESN'T TAKE MUCH, BUT IT SURELY DOES MUCH." MINDY L. MONTES

Your cells believe everything you think, feel, and say, so watch those thoughts, especially while rebounding. They are magnified in every cell. You can program-out old habits and thoughts, and program-in the new. Just repeat your affirmation over and over while you health bounce. This repeated impression becomes knowledge.

Rebound education can also be used to stimulate healing in the body. It is important, of course, to think positive, happy thoughts while rebounding, but you can direct specific messages to a certain area of the body to stimulate healing there.

Rebound education brings out the best in everyone. Self-esteem is greatly enhanced as you begin to feel greater vitality and improved overall health. Rebound education in our schools could be very valuable in enhancing the self-esteem of our children, developing leadership qualities.

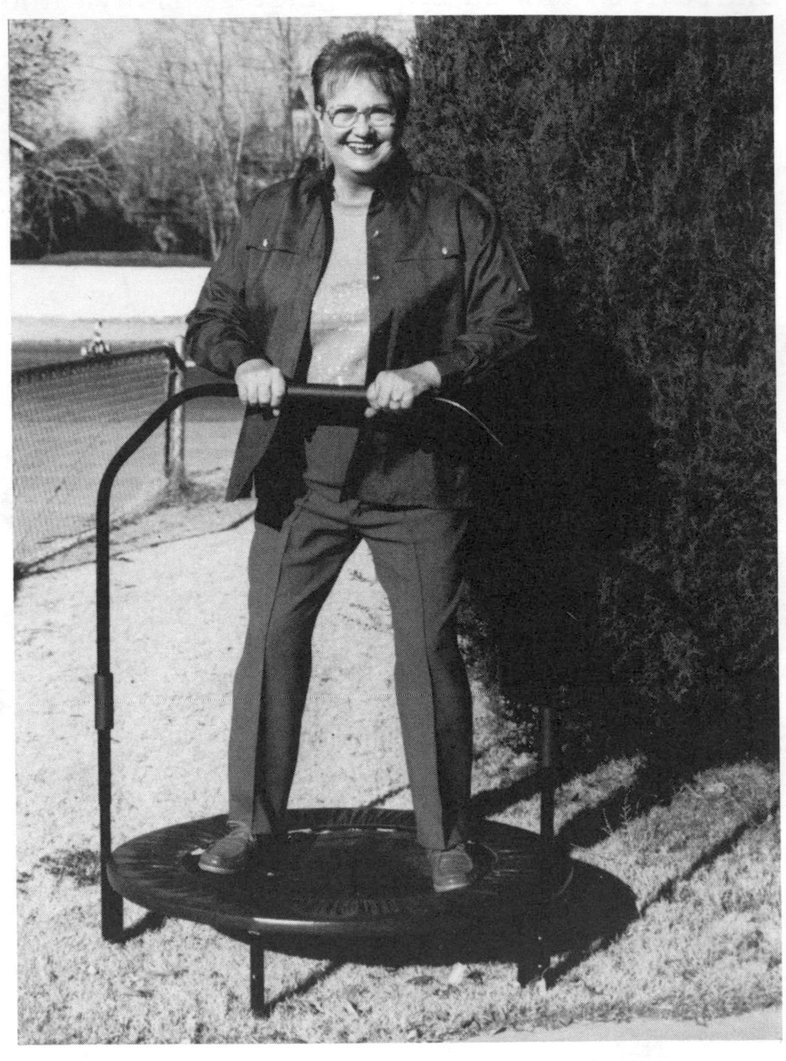

"YES! I HAVE BECOME A REBOUNDER ADDICT!!! WHY? BECAUSE I AM NO LONGER A COUCH POTATO. I ENJOY PLAYING BALL AND OTHER GAMES WITH MY GRANDCHILDREN AND THOSE OF MY FRIENDS. I AM DEEPLY GRATEFUL TO THE INVENTOR OF THE WONDERFUL PIECE OF EQUIPMENT CALLED THE REBOUNDER."

JOAN HEALD

CHAPTER VIII

Senior Rebounding

Rebound exercise is a very safe, healing, rejuvenating exercise for seniors. The constant pull of gravity on every cell of the body over the years, is a contributing factor in the aging and shrinking process. Rebounding reduces this effect because of its buoyancy. Bouncing with the stabilizer bar attached to the rebounder makes it possible to spring up slightly off the mat, so the body is weightless for a split second.

For seniors needing to increase circulation and cardiouascular strength, rebound exercise is extremely beneficial. Regular health bouncing strengthens bones and organs and improves the immune system.

If balance is a problem, the portable stabilizer bar should be added to your rebounder for security. Start off with easy bouncing for brief sessions of 1-2 minutes, or less, 4-5 times a day. Increase the length of your sessions as you feel ready.

I know folks who have worked up to bouncing and very light jogging for 10-15 minutes. Others love to bounce, jump, and jog. The important point is to start slowly, steadily increase your strength, and then lengthen your time. Then remember to be consistent.

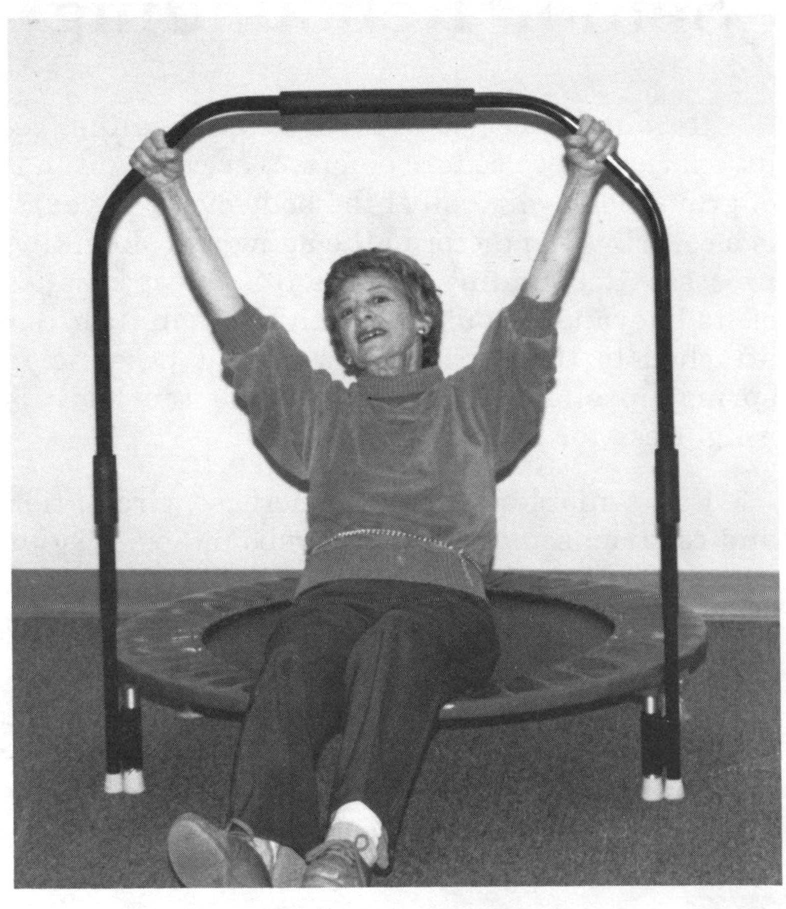

"AFTER A MONTH I (IN MY 70'S) AM ALREADY 'HOOKED' ON THIS ALSO AS AN INDOOR JOGGING MAT, VERY EASY ON THE KNEES WITH A PERSON'S LEAST EFFORT. I FIND IT A REAL FUN HEALTH AID, AND FOR BEST CIRCULATION. THE 'RETURNABLE' STABILIZER BAR ATTACHMENT LOANED FOR ME TO TRY, I SOON KNEW IT WAS TO BE MINE — AN IDEAL DEVICE STRENGTHENING MY SHOULDERS AND UPPER BODY. I'M GLAD TO SAY I'M HAPPILY ADDICTED TO THIS VERY SAFE 'BOUNCER'."

DIANE PALMER

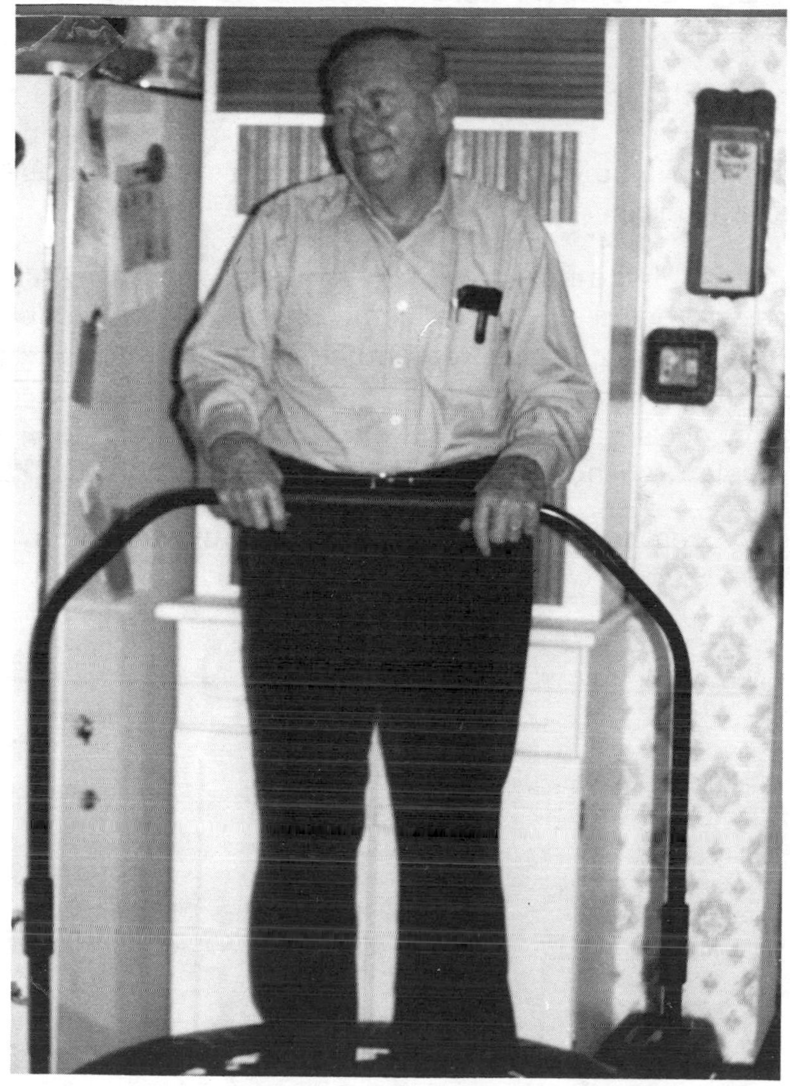

"BEFORE USING THE REBOUNDER, I COULDN'T WALK—I LITERALLY SHUFFLED AND STUMBLED MY WAY ALONG. NOW, I CAN WALK! MY BODY FEELS LIGHTER. MY SKIN USED TO BE PALE AND SALLOW, NOW IT'S A ROSY PINK. SINCE MORE BLOOD NOW GETS TO MY BRAIN, MY MEMORY IS IMPROVING EVERY DAY."

JAMES R. HEALD

Swing your arms down low to warm up, then bring them up to heart level for cardiovascular strength.

Hold on to the stabilizer bar with one hand, and stretch the other arm out and back, up and down to shoulder several times, then switch hands and exercise the other arm.

Hold the bar and kick your legs out in front as you bounce. Put on some music and do some light, slow jogging. Remember, moderation is the key to not overdoing it. Several short rebounding periods a day are more effective than one long session, without soreness or stress.

Breathe deeply and have fun on your rebounder!

CHAPTER IX

Rebounding With Disabilities and Handicaps

The powerful, shock-free benefits of rebound exercise, combined with its ease of application, makes it the ideal exercise for anyone, including those with severe disabilities and handicaps. Rebound exercise has even benefited people in wheel chairs. All that is needed is a little creativity in getting the person safely on the rebounder and then bouncing him.

A person in a wheel chair may just wheel up to the rebounder, lock the chair, then put his feet on the rebounder mat and have a buddy stand on the mat, straddling his feet, and do the health bounce.

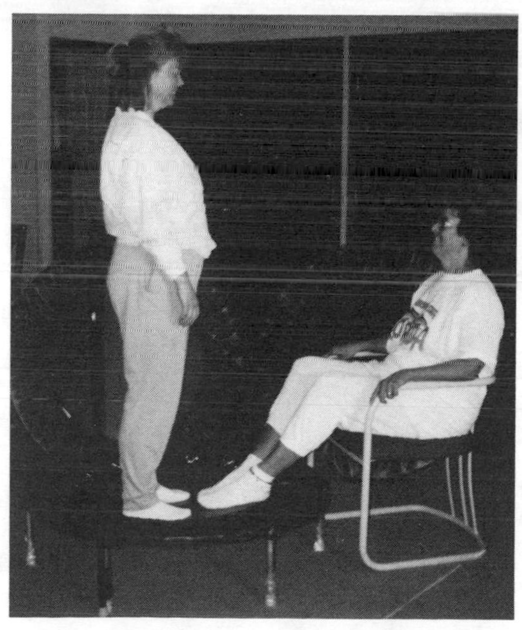

This exercises the cells of the lower part of the body, flushes lymph, and brings blood flow to each cell. To exercise the upper part of the body, the wheel chair person can then sit down on the rebounder mat, using the stabilizer bar if needed, and let the buddy stand behind him and do the health bounce again.

If a person can not stand or even sit up on the rebounder, then the buddy can help him lie down on the rebounder mat, stand and straddle him, and do the health bounce.

Those with weak or injured backs can health bounce with the stabilizer bar in place for very short sessions. Sometimes these sessions are only 15-20 seconds long, however they are very effec-

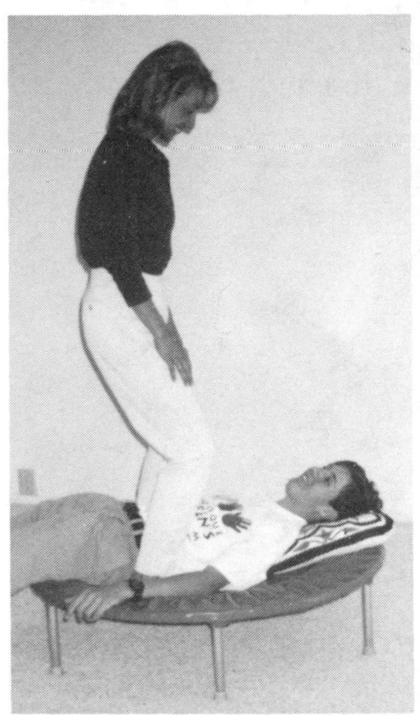

Peggy straddles Noah and gently bounces him 1-2 minutes, 4-5 times a day.

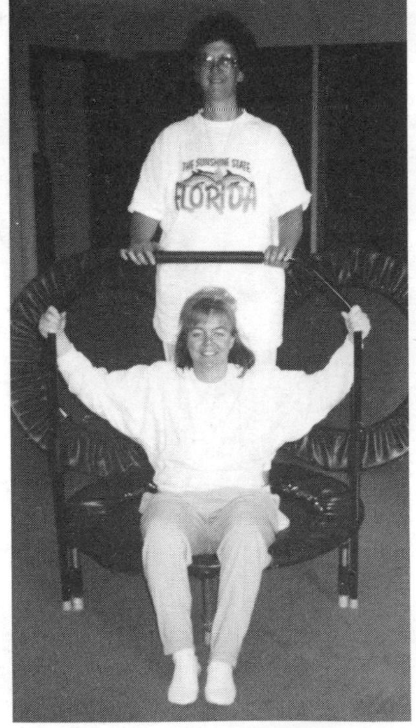

tive when done repeatedly throughout the day. After several days, depending on the severity of the weakness, the sessions can be increased, as strength and health are restored to each cell.

Sally health bounces with her feet on the mat for 15 seconds to 2 minutes, repeating this 4-5 times a day.

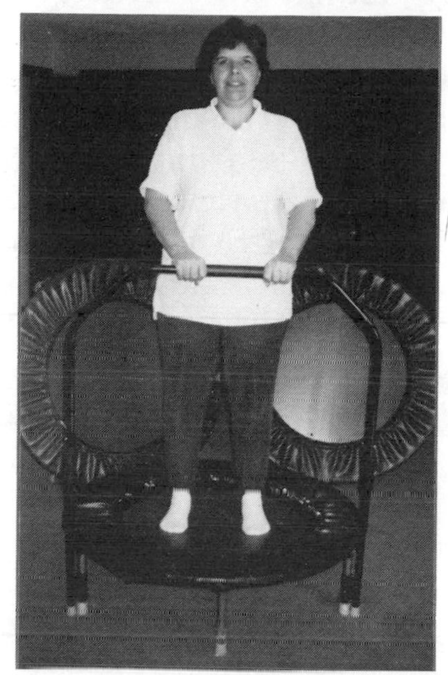

People with leg injuries, but with strength in their upper bodies, can sit on the rebounder mat with the stabilizer bar in place, and actually bounce

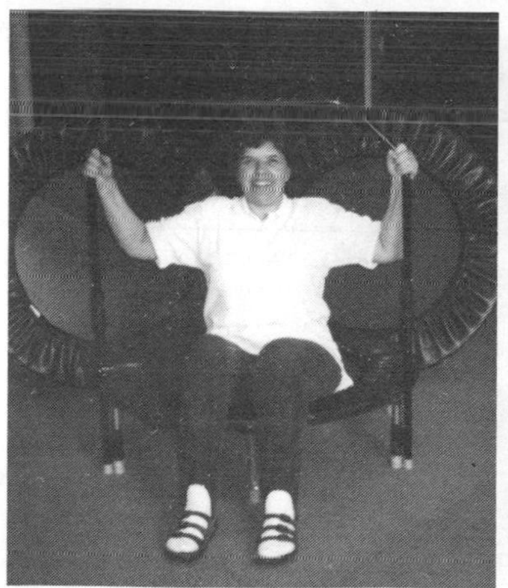

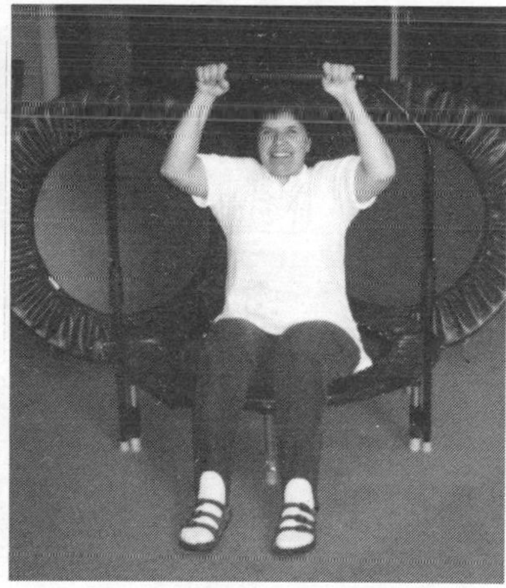

themselves by reaching up and gently pulling on the bar.

A person who has paralysis anywhere in the body just has to be creative about how to bounce, and decide whether a buddy is needed. Those able to stand up and bounce with the help of the stabilizer bar can health bounce for short sessions several times a day, paying attention to their threshold for pain or fatigue. If there is paralysis on one side of the body, that person could sit on the rebounder mat, reach up, and gently pull on the stabilizer bar with the unaffected arm, promoting the bouncing.

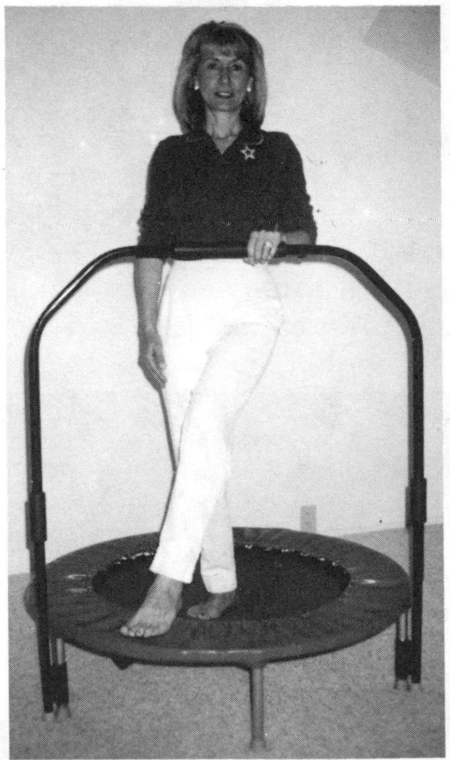

Peggy does a gentle front kick while holding the bar with her strong arm and relaxing the arm that needs healing.

By starting slowly, using the stabilizer bar, and being a little creative, rebounding's benefits can reach anyone, no matter what the condition.

Rebounding has been used for Physical therapy to promote balance, coordination, strength and healing, for many years. Be creative, add fun music, and bounce several times a day, increasing your time gradually, then expand your range of motion as you are able.

I have personally watched wheel chair patients, as well as those with leg, hip, knee, or back problems delight in health bouncing or being bounced by a buddy, getting cellular exercise, as

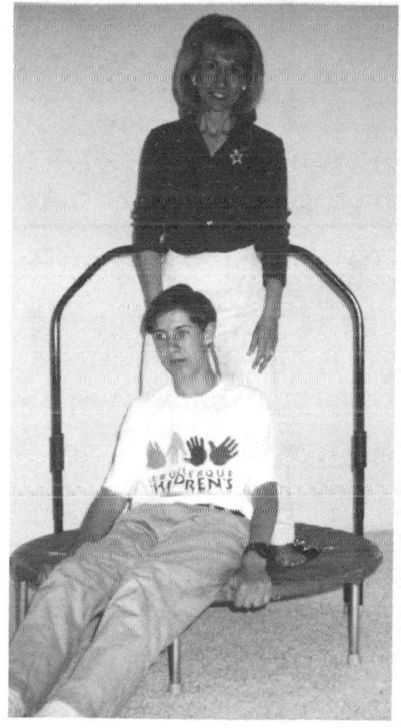

Noah relaxes against Peggy's legs as she provides support and gently health bounces him.

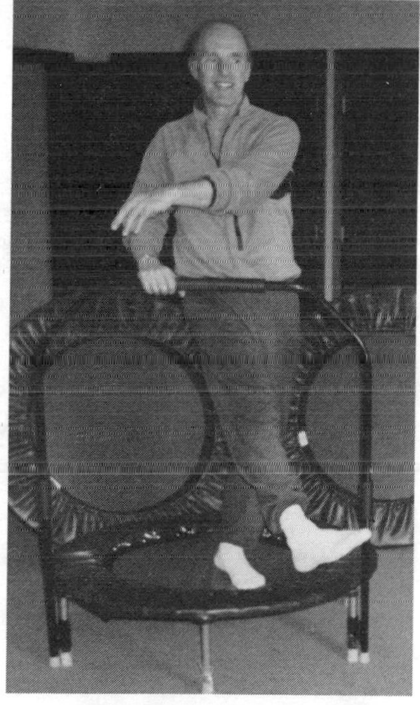

Bill does hand motions, alternating arms, enabling him to hold the stabilizer bar with the other hand.

they would otherwise not be able to do. I remember rehab patients taking pictures of each other as they tried out the Soft-bounce rebounder and stabilizer bar. Then there was the lady with one leg standing on the rebounder with the bar and bouncing for joy.

If you have a disability or a handicap, remember to find your threshold for pain or fatigue for your health bouncing sessions. You may feel a slight pain or pressure in the weak or affected area within a few seconds, rather than the normal 1-2 minutes for beginning bounces. That is the time to stop! Just note the amount of time that you had bounced before you felt the discomfort. That is your time threshold. It may be just a few seconds, but should not exceed 2 minutes for the beginning sessions.

Bounce for this threshold amount of time 4-5 times a day, every day, for the first week. You may gradually increase your time, however it is very effective to continue health bouncing for several sessions each day. The point is not to overdue. Remember that a beginning rebound session of 20-30 seconds is not unusual for someone with injuries or handicaps. When done safely and correctly, these extremely short sessions will gradually grow in length as tissue is rebuilt from the repeated cellular exercise. Persistence pays off!

Rebounding is safe, effective, and fun, and remember, can be used in any situation. Your health condition doesn't have to stop you from exercising. Now you can get the ideal exercise benefits to every single cell!

CHAPTER X

Celebration

Your body is a miracle. Celebrate it with nourishing, real food, clean water, rebound exercise, and loving thoughts. It will respond by throwing off toxins, negative emotions stored in cells, and unhealthy lifestyle habits, in order to become the purest temple possible for your Divine Spirit.

You are a sacred being - perfectly and wondrously made, awesome in design, and created by the same master artist who designed the solar system; the same creator who made the delicate roses and orchids, giant redwoods, intricate snowflakes, and sparkling diamonds. It's very apparent that "God don't make no junk," as the saying goes. You are a part of his magnificent creation, too!

We really don't know what we have the potential to accomplish on this earth. I'm sure you are aware of the fact that we use only a small percentage of our brain power. We also use a very small percentage of our life-power. With so many wonderful, natural tools for healing being given to us at this time, we are waking up to our potential as Children of God. That potential is awesome and unlimited.

Set a goal to make good health a way of life, not something you're struggling to attain. It is a step by step process,with you moving from higher level to higher level, joyfully.

Concentrating on basic, natural means of healing and maintaining health brings about a simplistic lifestyle. Rebound exercise is part of that simplicity, using natural forces that very powerfully cleanse and support your temple.

Enjoy every minute, every second, of the time you spend on your rebounder, and what an impact that will have on your health!

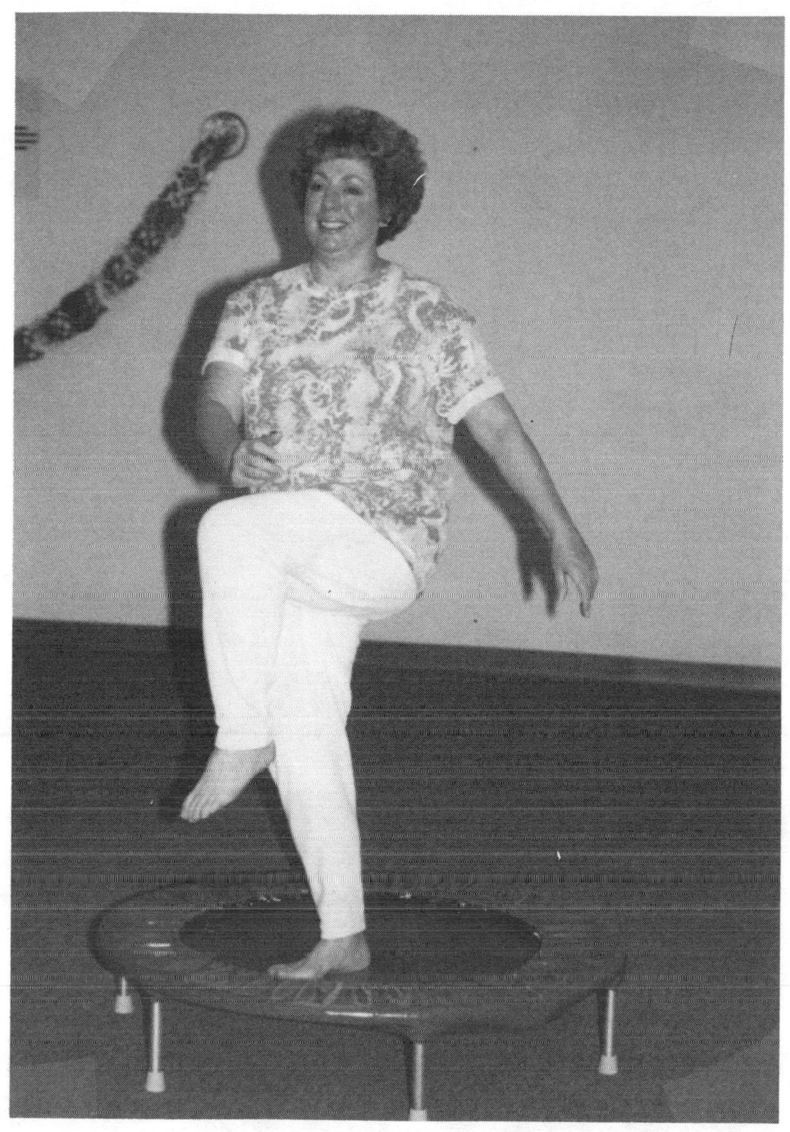

"REBOUNDING HAS BROUGHT ME AN INCREASE IN ENERGY, A DECREASE IN 'ACHES AND PAINS', AND JUST AN OVER ALL SENSE OF WELL BEING. WHAT WAS EXPECTED WAS AN IMPROVEMENT IN MY PHYSICAL HEALTH, BUT IT HAS ALSO TOUCHED MY SPIRITUAL BEING AND BROUGHT ME A WONDROUS FEELING OF PEACEFULNESS AND JOY." LINDA TROWBRIDGE

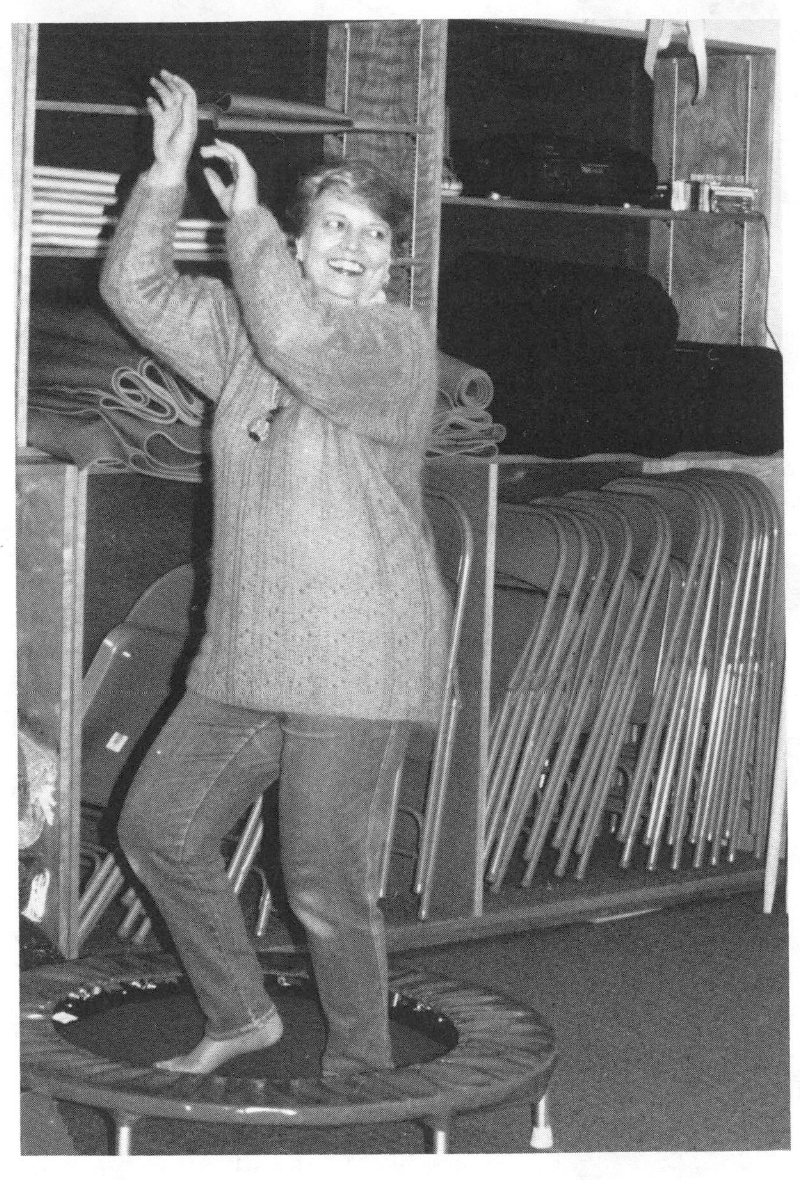

“CELEBRATION” BY JOYCE LOKEN

CHAPTER XI

Selecting a Unit

In 1984, 40 million rebound exercise units were sold. They were bought as toys, novelty items, or a fun exercise that few people understood. When mats stretched, frames bent, springs and legs broke on the cheaply made rebounders, these inferior units were tossed aside, and many of the manufacturers went out of business.

The old adage, "You get what you pay for," always rings true, but in choosing a rebounder, it is extremely important to look for quality construction because this exercise affects every cell in your body. An inferior mat made of nylon or canvas can split out or stretch. This could cause your weight to be thrown toward the middle of the mat, turning your ankles adversely, and putting strain on your spine.

Legs that screw on and off can be troublesome as threads wear thin. The springs on a rebounder are very important and should be resilient enough to supply bounce without stretching out of shape or breaking. An aluminum frame can bend or break.

I recommend American-made units made by NEEDAK Mfg. that are the highest quality rebounders on the market today, with the unique fold-up feature. These American-made units have a special Permatron® long-lasting mat that provides an invigorating bounce. The 36 high quality jumbo springs provide a buoyant bounce and longer life. The 40" heavy-duty steel frame has individual spring mounting pins to prevent frame wear.

Choose a stationary unit with spring-loaded folding legs or a completely portable rebounder that folds in half and fits in a carrying case. It is the only one of its kind.

The revolutionary Soft Bounce™ unit provides more buoyancy to promote healing of injuries, fun for seniors, or an invigorating workout for aerobics lovers.

For more information on these quality rebound units, see the order sheet at the end of this book.

Bounce in good health!

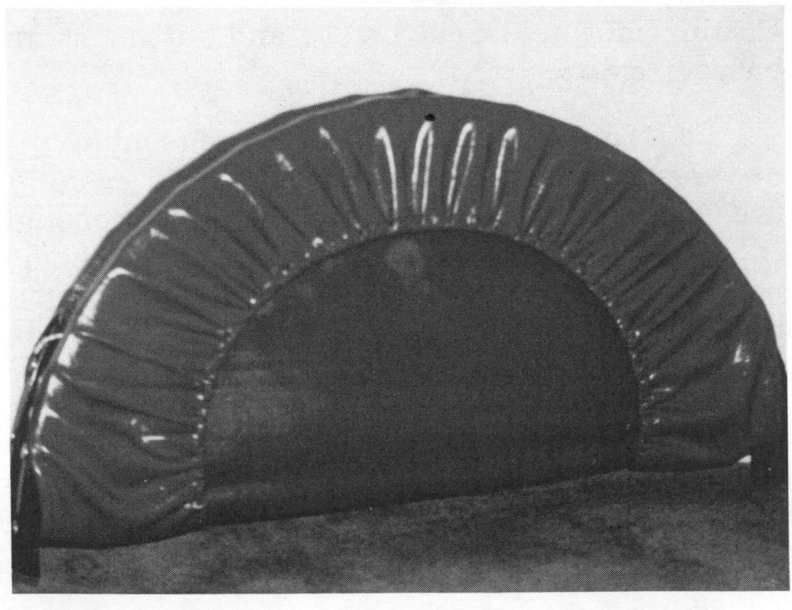

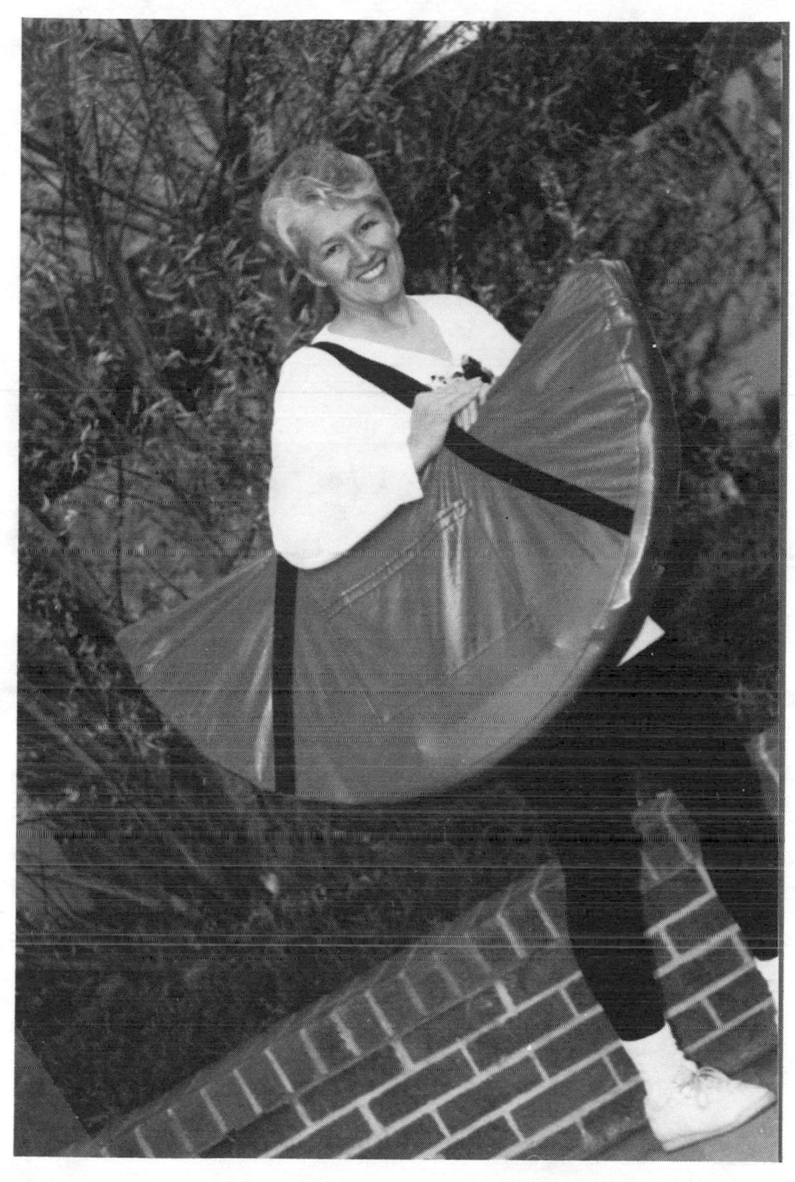

HAVE REBOUNDER, WILL TRAVEL.

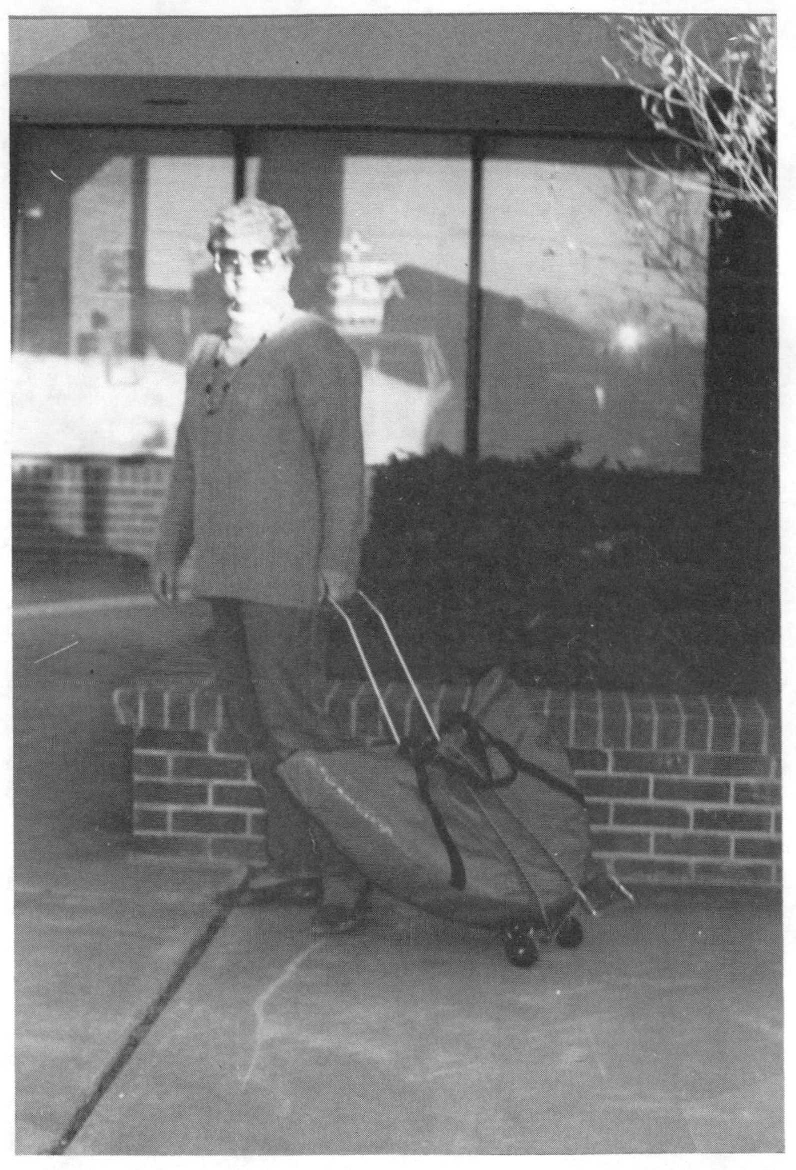

JOYCE IS READY FOR HER FLIGHT.

CHAPTER XII

A Rebound Album

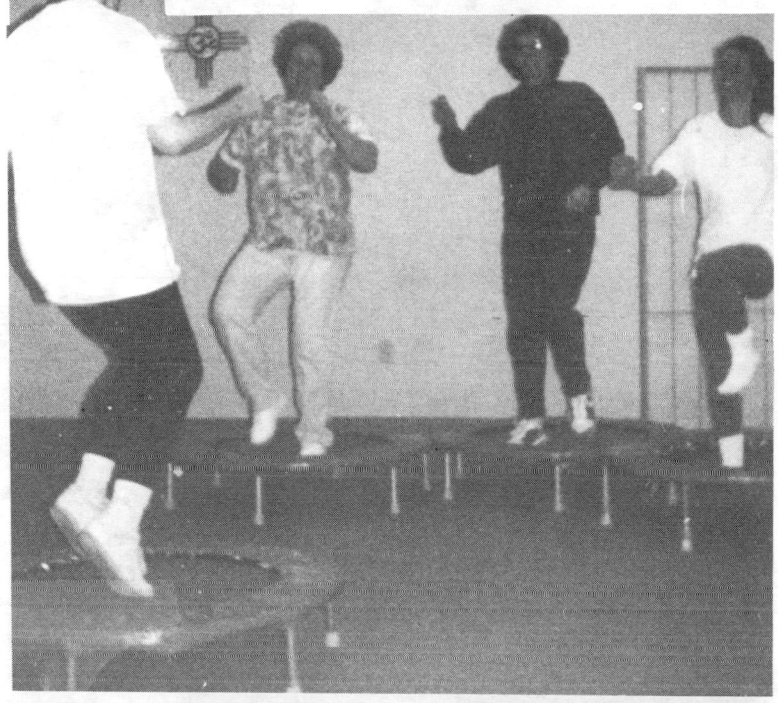

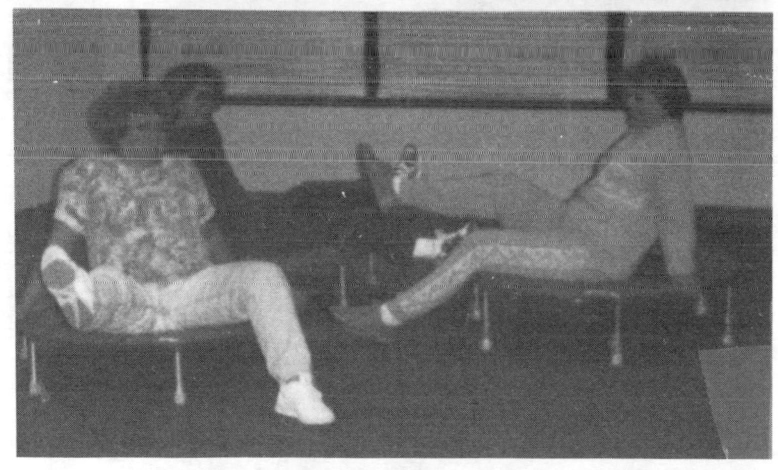

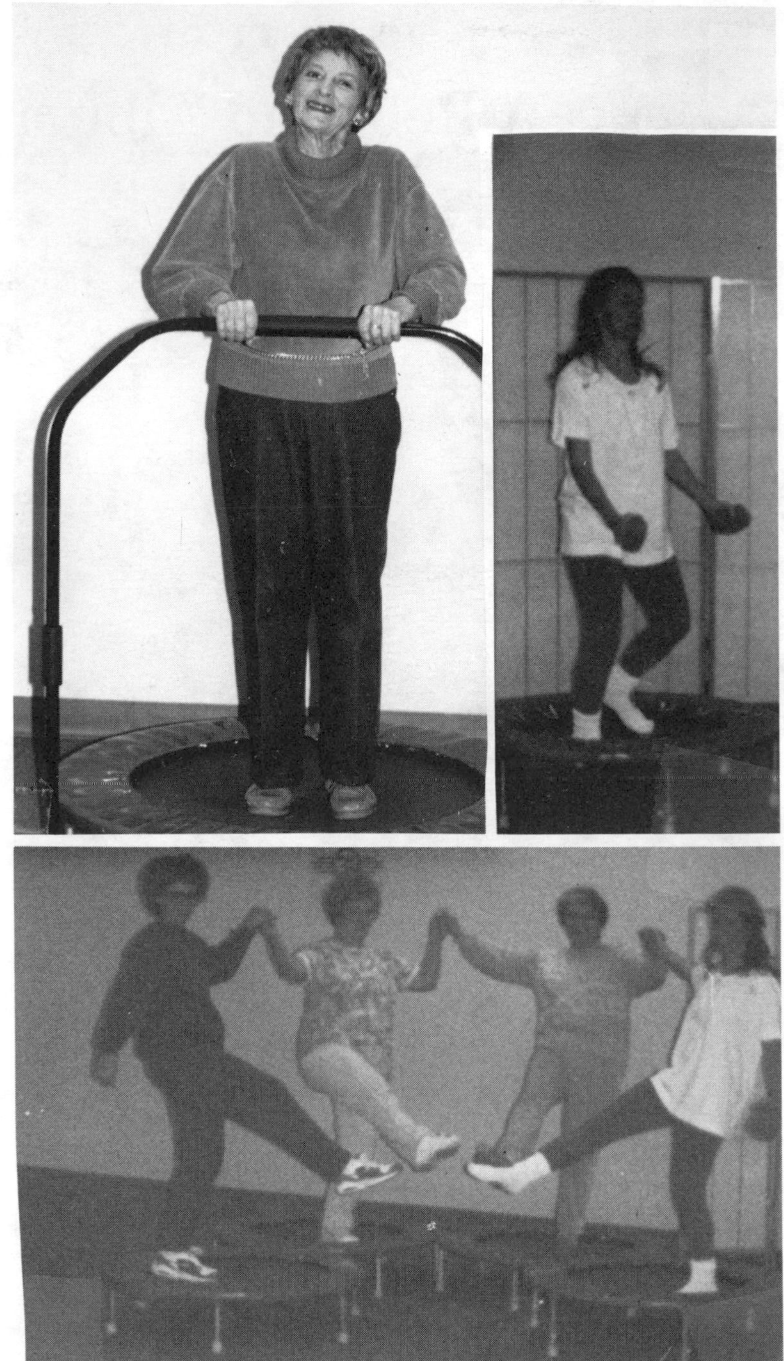

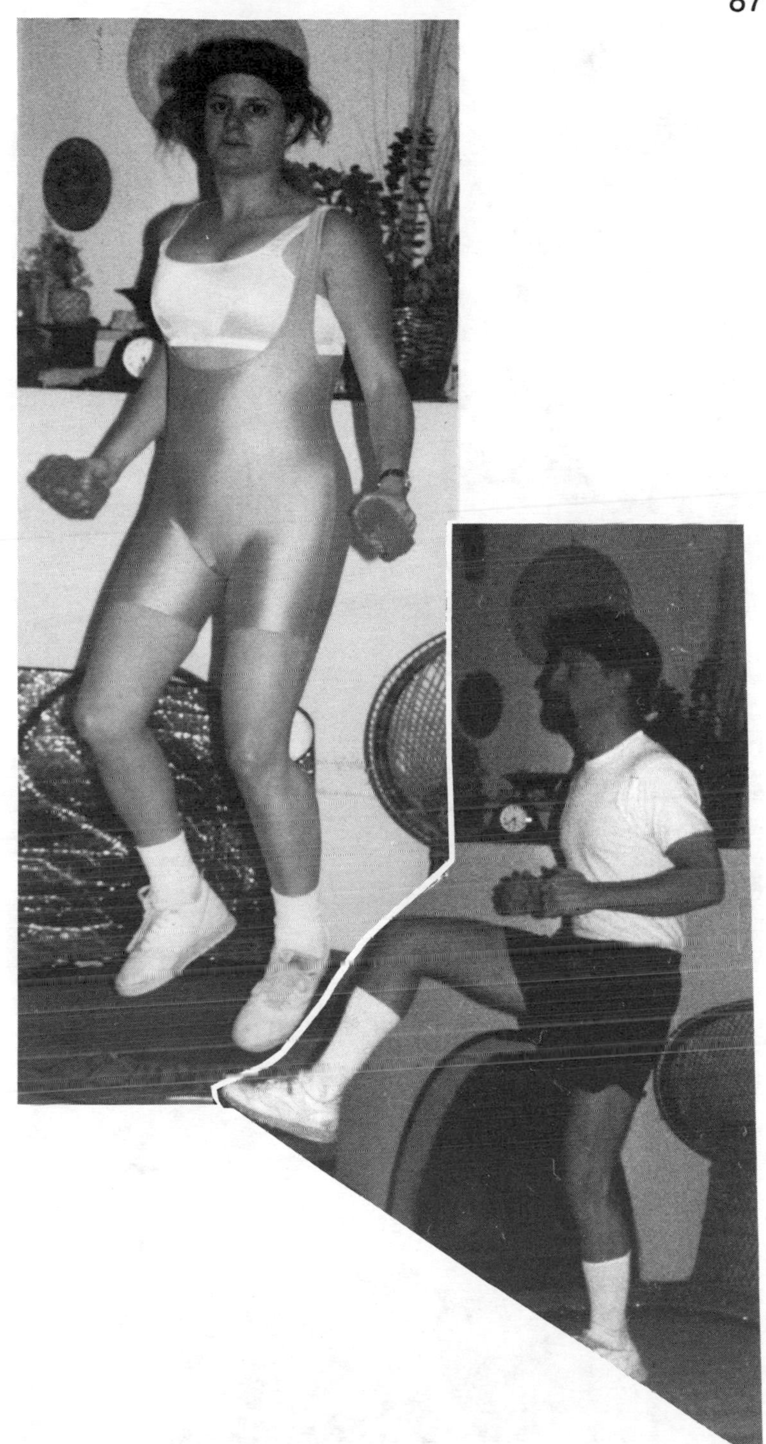

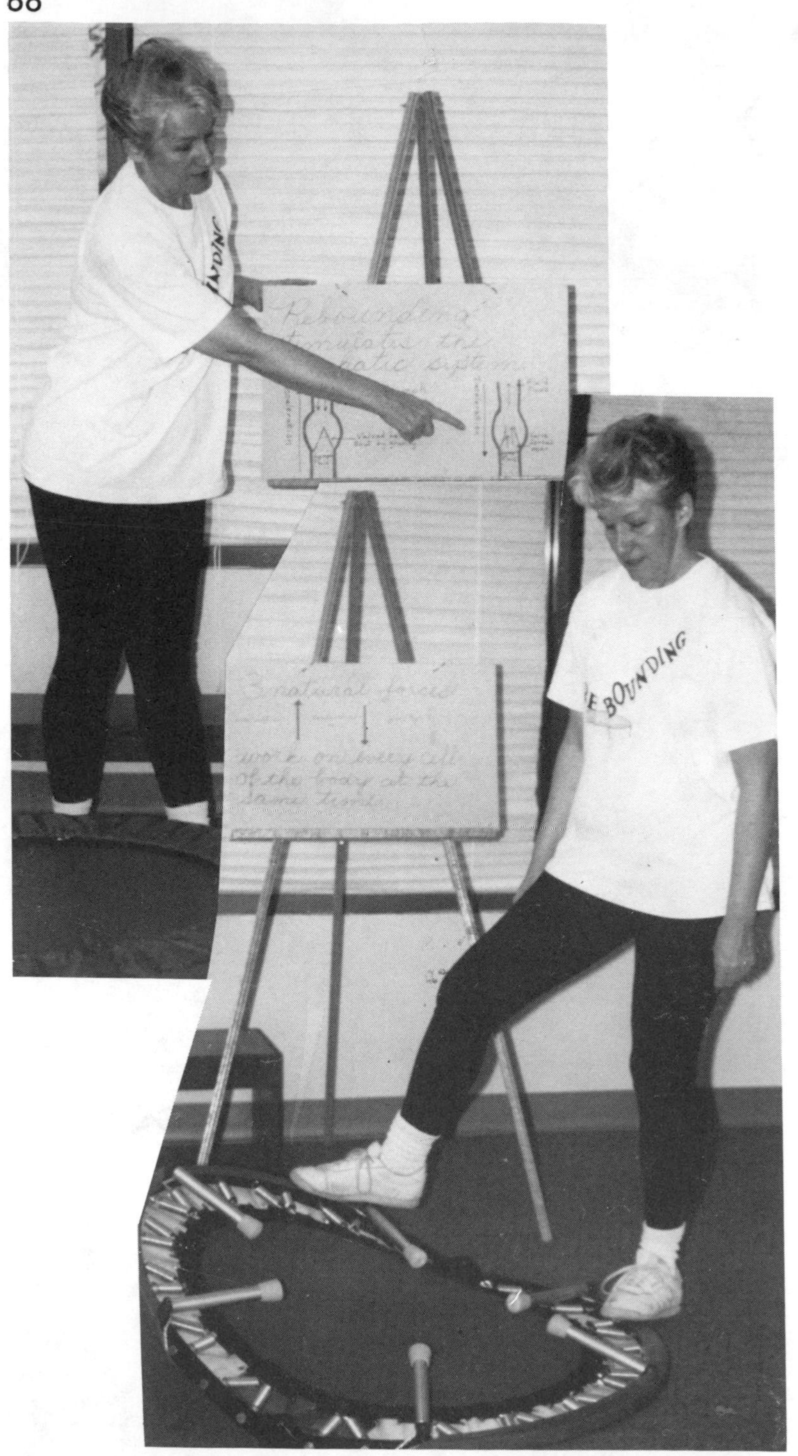
BOUNDING
3 natural forces

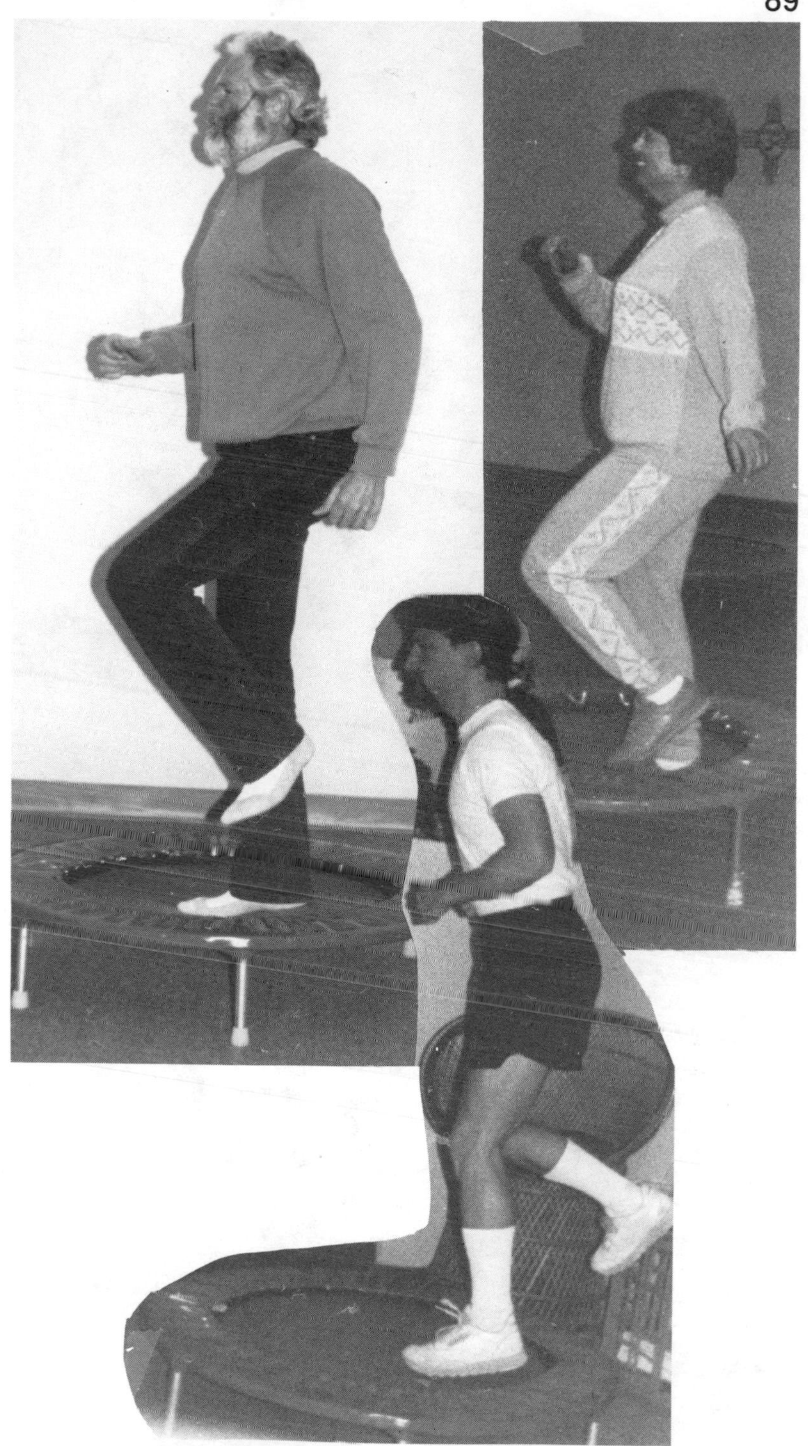

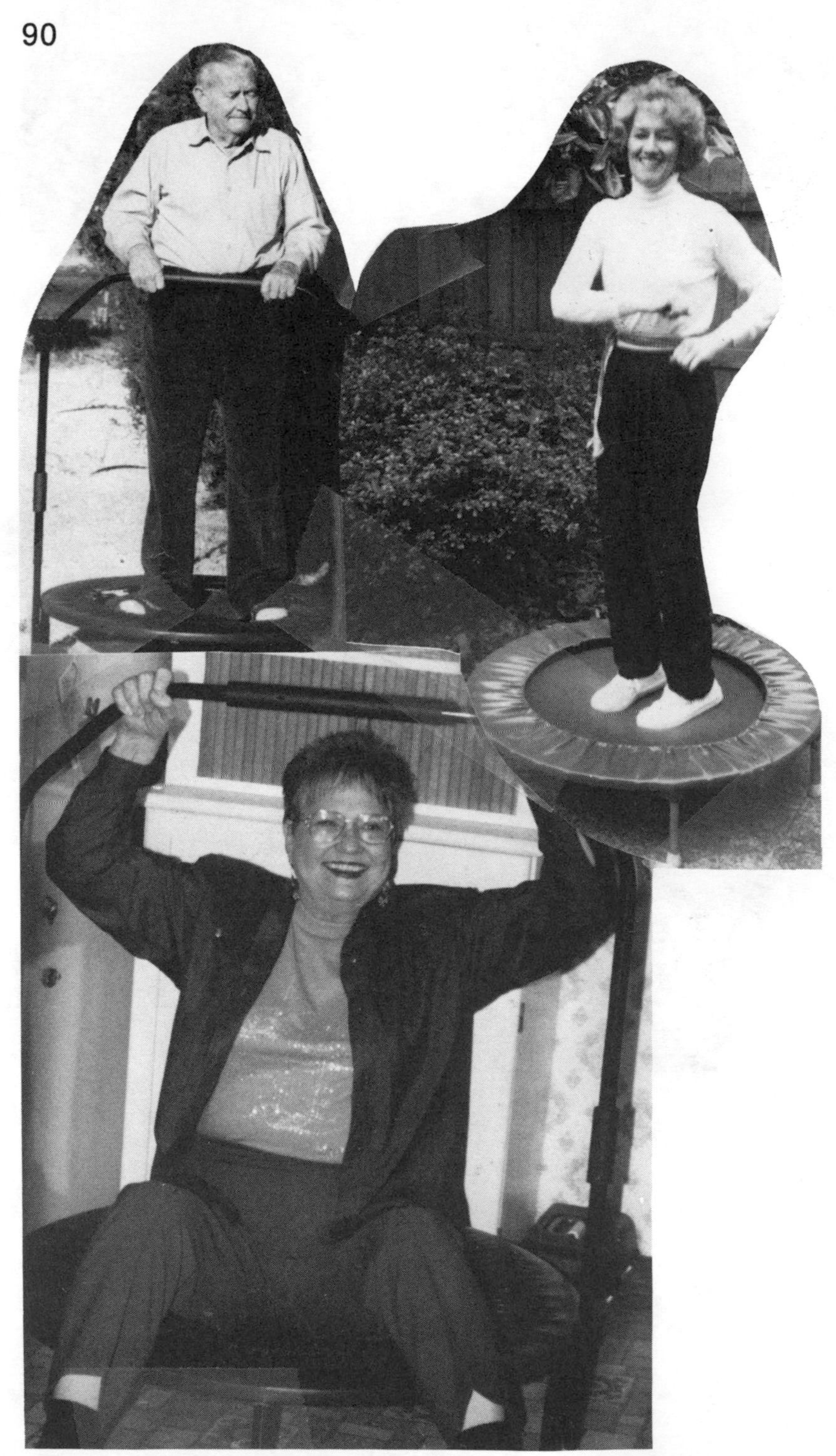

EVERYONE CAN REBOUND

Busy Mothers	Quick, stress-free exercise without going to the gym.
Executives	At home and at the office. Quick, energizing, mentally stimulating.
Children	Build balance, strength, coordination, and improve learning.
Seniors	Bounce for healing or health maintenance with stabilizer bar for balance and security.
Athletes	Improve strength, agility, endurance, and accuracy.
Aerobics Enthusiasts	Burn more calories, with less shock, more fun.
Invalids	Sit on the rebounder and bounce with stabilizer bar for support.
Injuries	Persons with knee, ankle or back injuries — a safe, shock-free, healing exercise.

SAMPLE PROGRAMS

Seniors and Beginners

	Health Bounce	Strength Bounce	Aerobic Bounce	Health Bounce	Times per day
Week 1	2 minutes				4 - 5
Week 2	1 minute		1 minute	1 minute	4
Week 3	1 minute	1 minute	2 minutes	1 minute	3 - 4
Week 4	1 minute	1 minute	3 minutes	1 minute	3

Beginning Aerobics

	Health Bounce	Strength Bounce	Aerobic Bounce	Health Bounce	Times per day
Week 1	1 minute		1 minute	1 minute	4 - 5
Week 2	1 minute	1 minute	5 minutes	1 minute	4
Week 3	1 minute	1 minute	10 minutes	1 minute	3
Week 4	1 minute	1 minute	30 - 40 minutes	1 minute	1

After the fourth week, you may add brief health bounces twice a day along with your aerobic workout.

VITAL HEALTH NEWS

A newsletter for body, mind and spirit with a back-to-basics approach to cellular health.

Linda's uplifting approach has inspired hundreds of individuals on their path to greater health and fulfillment for over twelve years. Enjoyment of greater health is now as close as your mailbox. Subscribe today, and each month be inspired by:

Rebound cellular exercise - creative routines, success stories, interviews about rebounding, senior news, educational rebound articles in ***Your Amazing Body section,*** new rebound product announcements, specials, and much more!

Food for your cells - Check ***The Nutrition Corner*** for vegetarian recipes, discussions with health care practitioners, the basics on internal cleansing, shopping tips, the truth about your food and your health, news about support products, and more.

Motivation and Inspiration - Recommended books and guidelines for taking charge of your health, lifestyle enhancement, all with motivational messages of truth and love that have made Linda's newsletter grow in popularity year after year!

"Your monthly newsletter is like a ray of sunshine in my life" **N. Carolina**	***Your new format is just great. I just love it and don't want to miss an issue!"*** **Alberta, Canada**
"Your newsletters are great. I don't want to miss an issue!" **Wisconsin**	***"Your newsletter is very informative."*** **Florida**

Subscribe today to this unique and timely newsletter!

[ ] **1-year** subscription: **$28.00** In Canada **$36.00**
[ ] **2-year** subscription: **$44.00** In Canada **$55.00**
[ ] **3-year** subscription: **$56.00** In Canada **$77.00**

(Get one year free with three!)

Name ______________________ Phone __________

Address ______________________________

City ______________________ State _____ Zip __________

Mail to:
The Vitally Yours Center, 750 Boyce St., Urbana, OH 43078
Phone orders: 937-484-8206 Visa, MC, Discover cards, checks or money orders in U.S. funds.

BOUNCE BEFORE YOU JUMP

An Introduction to Rebound Movement

by Linda Brooks, Certified Reboundologist

Bounce Before You Jump is a great introductory video for the first time rebounder. Linda Brooks, author of Rebounding to Better Health will teach you:

How to stand on the rebounder
Proper rebound posture
How to safely and effectively bounce, jump, and do aerobic moves
When to utilize each movement
Rebounding for therapy, weight loss, seniors, sports, and aerobics
How to use the stabilizing bar effectively

Create routines that fit your needs and enjoyment. Linda also provides short workouts for the beginner, intermediate and advanced student.

Bounce Before You Jump
by Linda Brooks,
approx. 80 Minutes

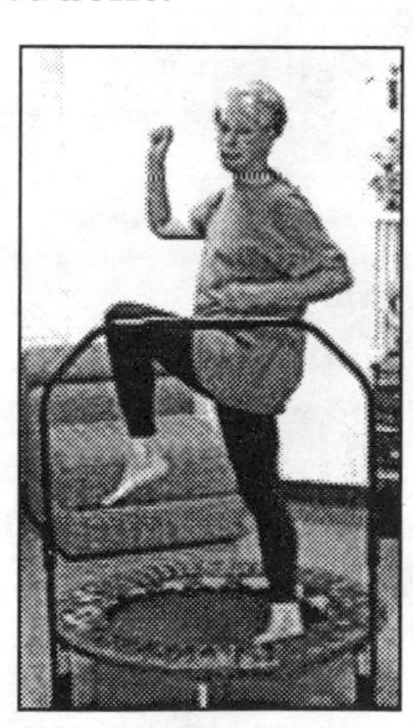

This and many other titles are available through your
Needak® dealer

or call

1-800-232-5762
1-402-336-4083

THE IMMUNE SYSTEM VIDEO

Al Carter is known for his informative and entertaining presentation of the Healthy Cell Concept. Learn

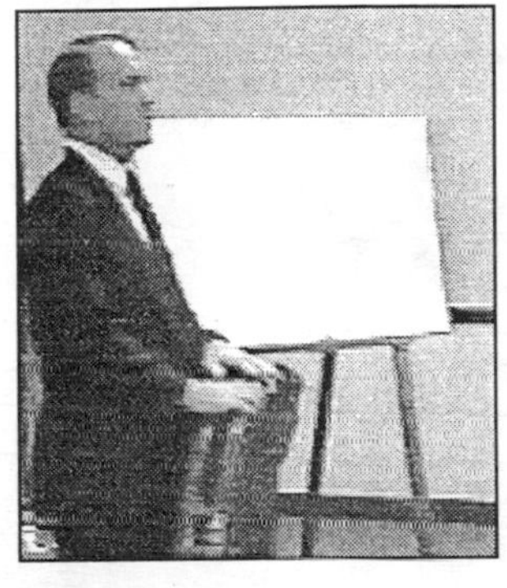

about your immune system-how it functions to keep you healthy and disease free. You will also learn about the importance of good foods, clean water, and rebound exercise in supporting your immune system.

The information contained on this video is pure dynamite. You will gain a greater appreciation of your body and how to maintain your good health. You will demand that your friends and family view it as well.

The Immune System by Albert Carter,
approx. 45 minutes.

This and many other video titles are
available through your
Needak® dealer

or call

1-800-232-5762
1-402-336-4083

Get all of the details about the popular URBAN REBOUNDING program!

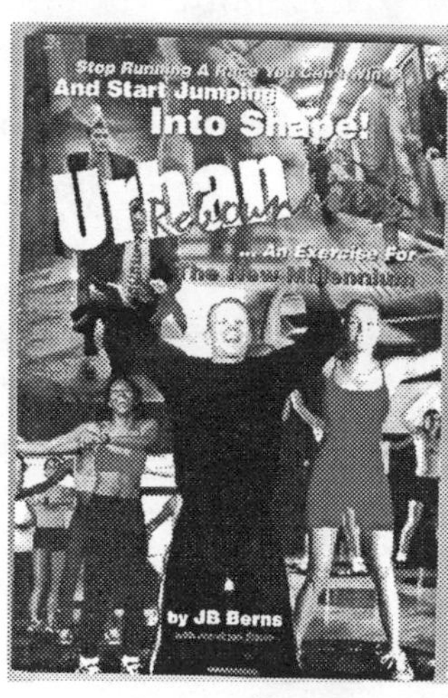

J. B. Berns, the developer of the Urban Rebounding system, explains how the program evolved and provides support information into the benefits of rebounding. The book provides details into the various movements done in the classes. This book is THE companion volume to the Urban Rebounding class.

This and many other titles are available
through your
Needak® dealer

or call

1-800-232-5762
1-402-336-4083